How to Correctly Answer EKG and Arrhythmia Questions

For Medical Students and Doctors Preparing for USMLE Step 1, Step 2 CK, and Step 3

Copyright page:

Notice: The author of this book has taken care to make certain that the recommendations for patient management and use of drugs are correct and compatible with the standards generally accepted at the time of publication. As any new information becomes available, changes in treatment and use of drugs are inevitable. The reader is advised to carefully consult the instructions and information material included in the package insert of each drug or therapeutic agent before administration. The author and publisher disclaim any liability, loss, injury or damage incurred as a consequence, directly or indirectly, of the use and application of any of the contents of this book.

Copyright © 2024 by Marks Medical Concepts LLC

All rights reserved. This book is protected by copyright. No part of it may be reproduced, stored in a retrieval system, or transmitted in any form or by any means, electronic, mechanical, photocopying, recording, or otherwise, without written permission from the copyright owner, except for the use of a brief quotation in a book review.

For rights and permissions, please email:
marksmedicalconcepts@gmail.com

ISBN-13: 979-8-218-43903-3

FREE BONUS BOOK

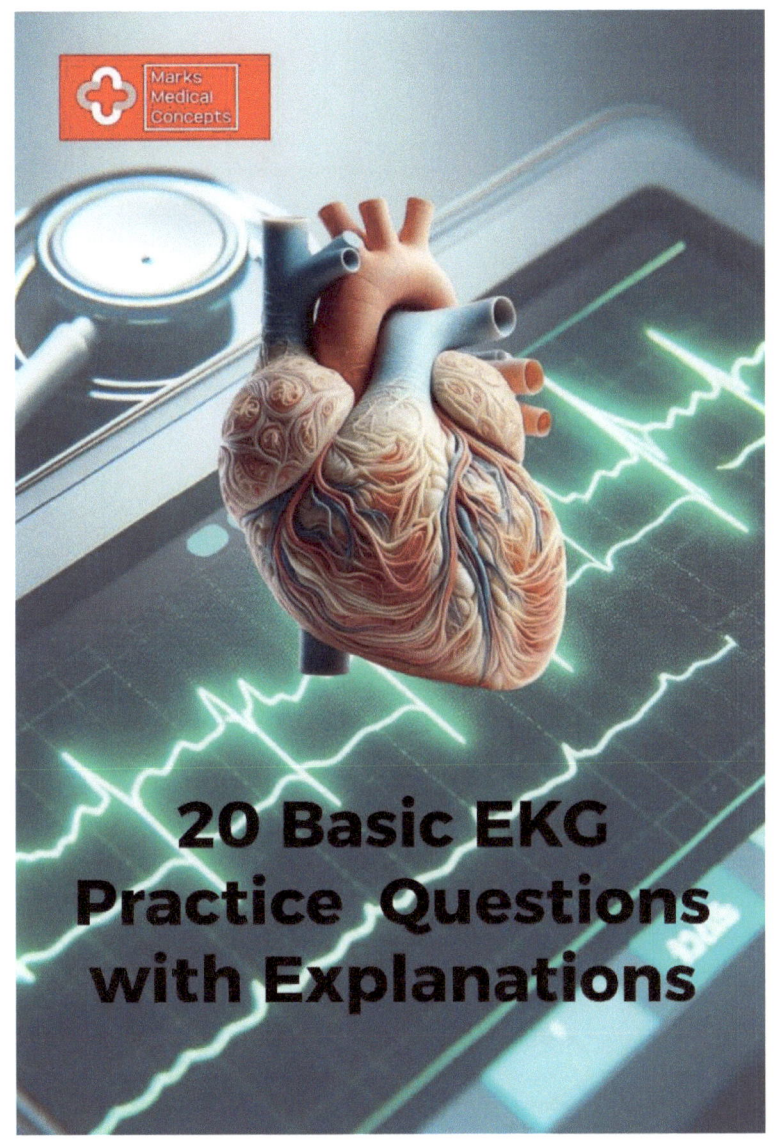

FREE DOWNLOAD – Just visit:
www.marksmedicalconcepts.com/download

TABLE OF CONTENT

Introduction..VI

Dedication..VII

Chapter 1: Question break down..1

Chapter 2: EKG foundations..6
  I. Cardiac Physiology
  II. Pacemakers
  III. Cardiac Anatomy
  IV. Understanding the EKG strip
  V. Causes of Changes in EKG Intervals and Durations

Chapter 3: Understanding Rate and Rhythm..10
  I. Rate
  II. Rhythm

Chapter 4: The Five Steps Used To Interpret Any EKG...12

Chapter 5: Arrhythmias..13
  I. Classification of Arrhythmias
  II. Tachycardia + Regular Arrhythmias
    a. Ventricular Tachycardia..14
    b. Wolff Parkinson White Syndrome..18
    c. Atrial Flutter..20
    d. Sinus Tachycardia..24
    e. Supraventricular Tachycardia..26
  III. Tachycardia + Irregular Arrhythmias
    a. Torsades de pointes..28
    b. Ventricular Fibrillation..30
    c. Multi-Focal Atrial Tachycardia..34
    d. Atrial Fibrillation...36
  IV. Bradycardia + Regular Arrhythmias
    a. Sinus Bradycardia..40
    b. First Degree Heart Block...42
    c. Third Degree Heart Block..44
  V. Bradycardia + Irregular Arrhythmias
    a. Second Degree Type 1 Heart Block...46
    b. Second Degree Type 2 Heart Block...48
  VI. Normal rate + Irregular Arrhythmias
    a. Wandering Pacemaker..50
  VII. Ectopic beats
    a. Premature Atrial Contractions..52
    b. Premature ventricular Contractions...53
  VIII. Other EKG findings
    a. Congenital Long QT Syndrome...54
    b. Hypothermia (Osborne Wave)..56
    c. Electrolyte Disorders..57
    d. Asystole..58
    e. Pulseless Electrical Activity..60
    f. Electrical Alternans..62
    g. Pulmonary Embolism...64
    h. ST Elevation/ Depression...66

Abbreviations and Symbols..80
Index...81

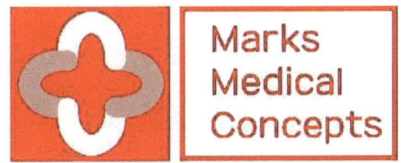

Check out more educational products and join our newsletter at

www.marksmedicalconcepts.com/USMLE

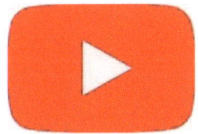

Watch our new videos on

Marks Medical USMLE

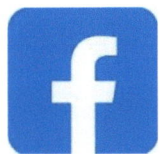

Follow us on Facebook at

Marks Medical USMLE

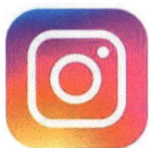

Follow us on Instagram at

Marks Medical USMLE

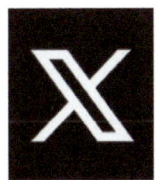

Follow us on X at

Marks Medical USMLE

Introduction

EKG questions can be either a gentle breeze or a storm, depending on your readiness. They might make you elicit a huge smile during your exam or set off an impromptu sweat session. This powerful book was specifically made to promote confidence when attempting EKG questions. There are so many reasons why this book is special, such as:

1. Simplicity:

Remember the saying, "True elegance is in simplicity"? Well, consider this book the embodiment of that wisdom. Each section is crafted with clarity, ensuring comprehension and long-term retention. The information here is straightforward and crystal-clear.

2. Quick comprehension:

Busy med student or physician? We get it. This book was written for the information to be quickly comprehended. Read it swiftly, absorb the essentials, and still have time for other exam topics.

3. Interpret any arrhythmia quickly:

Using this book, you will learn how to analyze any EKG quickly and efficiently with the 5-step process. This will help you make an accurate diagnosis while answering questions.

4. All the EKGs you will need:

Each arrhythmia has both a 6-second single-strip EKG and a 12-lead EKG. These EKGs will provide you with a strong foundation for EKG pattern recognition.

5. Colorful and memorable images:

The images and EKGs come alive with clarity. The vibrant colors are like memory magic, which helps to promote recall even when you become a seasoned physician a decade from now.

6. Lifelong companion:

This isn't just a book, it's a lifelong companion. Even after you have successfully passed all your exams, keep this book handy. Mastering EKGs isn't just about exams, it's about becoming the best physician you can be. This wonderful book will provide you with all the necessary information for interpreting EKGs.

Dedication

This book is dedicated to my brother Emeka Anombem, the first friend I ever knew and the best teammate I could ever ask for. You have always been a constant source of encouragement and are the reason I believe anything is possible. This book wouldn't exist without your unwavering support. Also, I dedicate this book to my beloved wife and our precious son. Your never ending support and deep understanding have been the very heartbeat of my inspiration and the driving force behind every word penned in this book. I also dedicate this book to my late father and loving mother, who provided me with a loving home and a solid foundation to achieve great things. Finally, I dedicate this book to all medical students striving to become physicians so they can heal patients and make the world a better place.

THIS PAGE INTENTIONALLY LEFT BLANK

CHAPTER 1:
QUESTION BREAK DOWN

Question 1:
A 64-year-old man presents to the ER with complaints of palpitation, which started 30 minutes earlier. He has a history of hypertension and diabetes, which both started about ten years ago. He has smoked one pack of cigarettes daily for the past 20 years. Upon examination, he was sweating, and his pulse rate was 190 BPM. EKG showed an arrhythmia with a narrow QRS and regular rhythm. What is the diagnosis?
   A. Ventricular tachycardia
   B. Supraventricular tachycardia
   C. Ventricular Fibrillation
   D. Wolff Parkinson White syndrome

Question 1 answer is B. Supraventricular tachycardia. The diagnosis for this patient is Supraventricular tachycardia (SVT) because the QRS is narrow, the rhythm is regular, and the heart rate is greater than 100 BPM. All the other options for this question have wide QRS complexes, SVT is the only option with a narrow QRS complex.

A TYPICAL ARRHYTHMIA QUESTION HAS THE FOLLOWING COMPONENTS:

Typical history findings:

Age: Patients with Arrhythmias are usually Middle-aged or elderly—for example, A 64-year-old man.

ER: Patients with arrhythmias usually present at the ER.

History of Heart disorder: Patients with arrhythmias usually have a history of a heart condition—for example, Myocardial infarction history or cardiomyopathy.

Comorbidities: Patients with arrhythmia usually have **(HH SODA) H**TN, **H**yperlipidemia, **S**moker, **O**besity, **D**iabetes, **A**ge greater than 35 years.
+
Typical arrhythmia clinical features: LDL PP
L Lightheadedness
D Dizziness
L Loss of consciousness (LOC)
+
P Palpitation
P Pulse: Tachycardia, bradycardia, regular rhythm or irregular rhythm
+
Typical EKG findings:
Rate: Bradycardia, normal or tachycardia
Rhythm: regular or irregular
P wave: Present, absent or inverted
PR interval: increased or decreased
QRS duration: wide or narrow

TYPES OF EKG QUESTIONS:
There are three types of EKG questions:
   1. EKG question with a **12-lead EKG strip**
   2. EKG question with a **Single lead EKG strip**
   3. EKG question with **No EKG strip**

1. <u>**EKG question with a 12-lead EKG strip:**</u>

Here, you are given a 12-lead EKG strip with a question.

<u>Question 2:</u>

A 22-year-old tall Caucasian male came into the ER with palpitation. An EKG was done, which is shown below. What is the diagnosis?

A. Atrial fibrillation
B. Wolff Parkinson white syndrome
C. Normal sinus rhythm

(Check at the beginning of the next page for the answer)

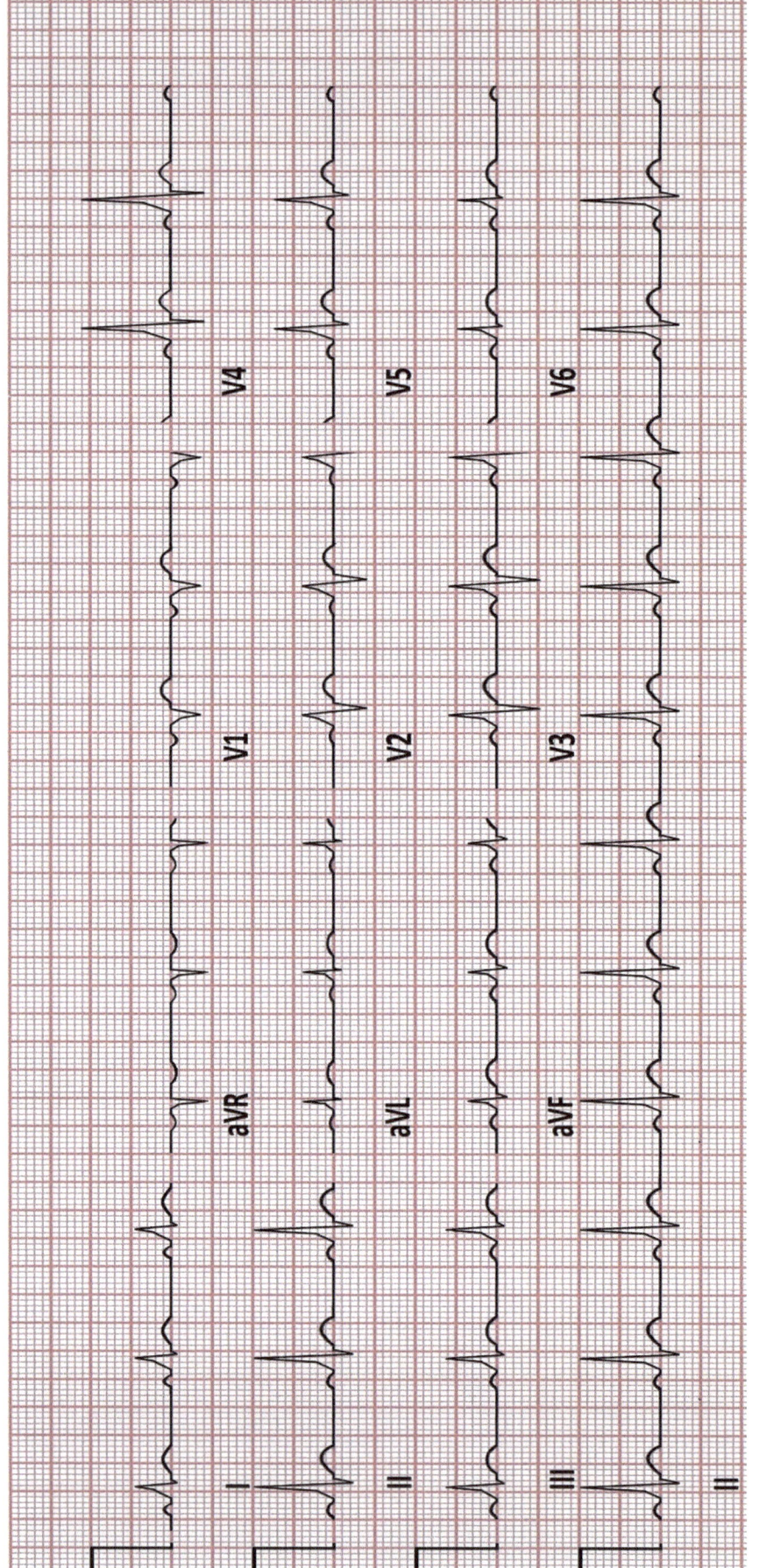

Question 2 answer: B. Wolff Parkinson White syndrome. On the 12-lead EKG, you can see the following:
- The delta waves
- Short PR interval
- Classic presentation of a tall Caucasian male with palpitation

2. **EKG question with a Single lead EKG strip:**

In this type of question, you are given a single lead EKG strip and a question.

Question 3:

A 57-year-old female came into the ER with complaints of palpitation. An EKG was done, which is shown below. What is the diagnosis?

A. Atrial fibrillation
B. Multifocal atrial tachycardia
C. Sinus tachycardia

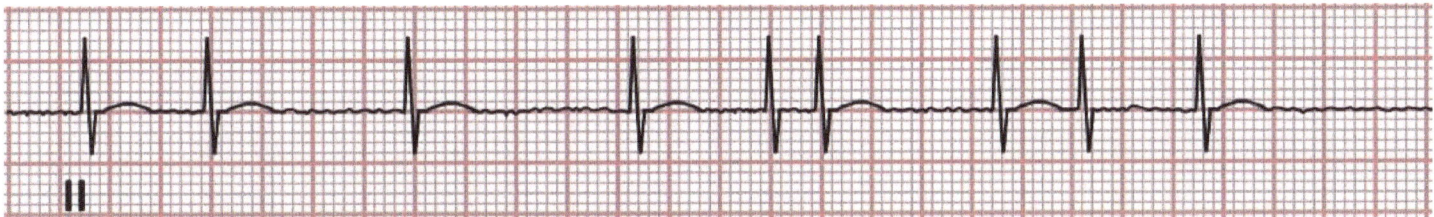

Question 3 answer: A. Atrial fibrillation. On the single lead EKG, you can see the following:
- No P waves are present. Only Fibrillary waves
- Rhythm is irregular
- Narrow QRS duration less than 80 ms

3. **EKG question with NO EKG strip:**

In this type of question, you may be given a clinical vignette without an EKG strip attached to the question. Because these questions do not provide you with an EKG strip, it is very important for you to learn how to classify arrhythmias. You have to know which arrhythmias are regular or irregular, and which ones have a wide or narrow QRS. An example of this type of question is shown below.

Question 4:

A 42-year-old man comes to the ER complaining of palpitations and lightheadedness. His pulse is regular on palpation. An EKG done showed a rhythm with a narrow QRS. Which of the following is the likely diagnosis?

A. Atrial fibrillation
B. Ventricular fibrillation
C. Torsades de pointes
D. Atrial flutter

Question 4 Answer: D Atrial flutter. The answer is simple because it is the only arrhythmia listed in the option with a regular rhythm and a narrow QRS.

THE UNSTABLE PATIENT QUESTION:

For any patient with an arrhythmia and unstable clinical features, regardless of the type of arrhythmia, synchronized cardioversion is the recommended treatment for these patients.

The four clinical features that indicate a patient is unstable, which you must look for in every arrhythmia question are:
ABCD
A AMS (Altered Mental Status)
B BP ↓ (Hypotension)
C Chest pain
D Dyspnea (Shortness of breath)

Treatment of an unstable patient with arrhythmias:

> Unstable Clinical Features: **(ABCD)**
> **A** AMS (Altered Mental Status)
> **B** BP ↓ (Hypotension)
> **C** Chest pain
> **D** Dyspnea (Shortness of breath)

↓

1. If any of the unstable symptoms above are present
The treatment is **synchronized cardioversion**
This is the only time you will ever use synchronized cardioversion to treat a patient. If you see it as an option in any other question where the patient is stable, **that option is always wrong.**

2. If all the unstable symptoms above are absent:
The treatment is **specific for that particular arrhythmia**

SYNCHRONISED MAN

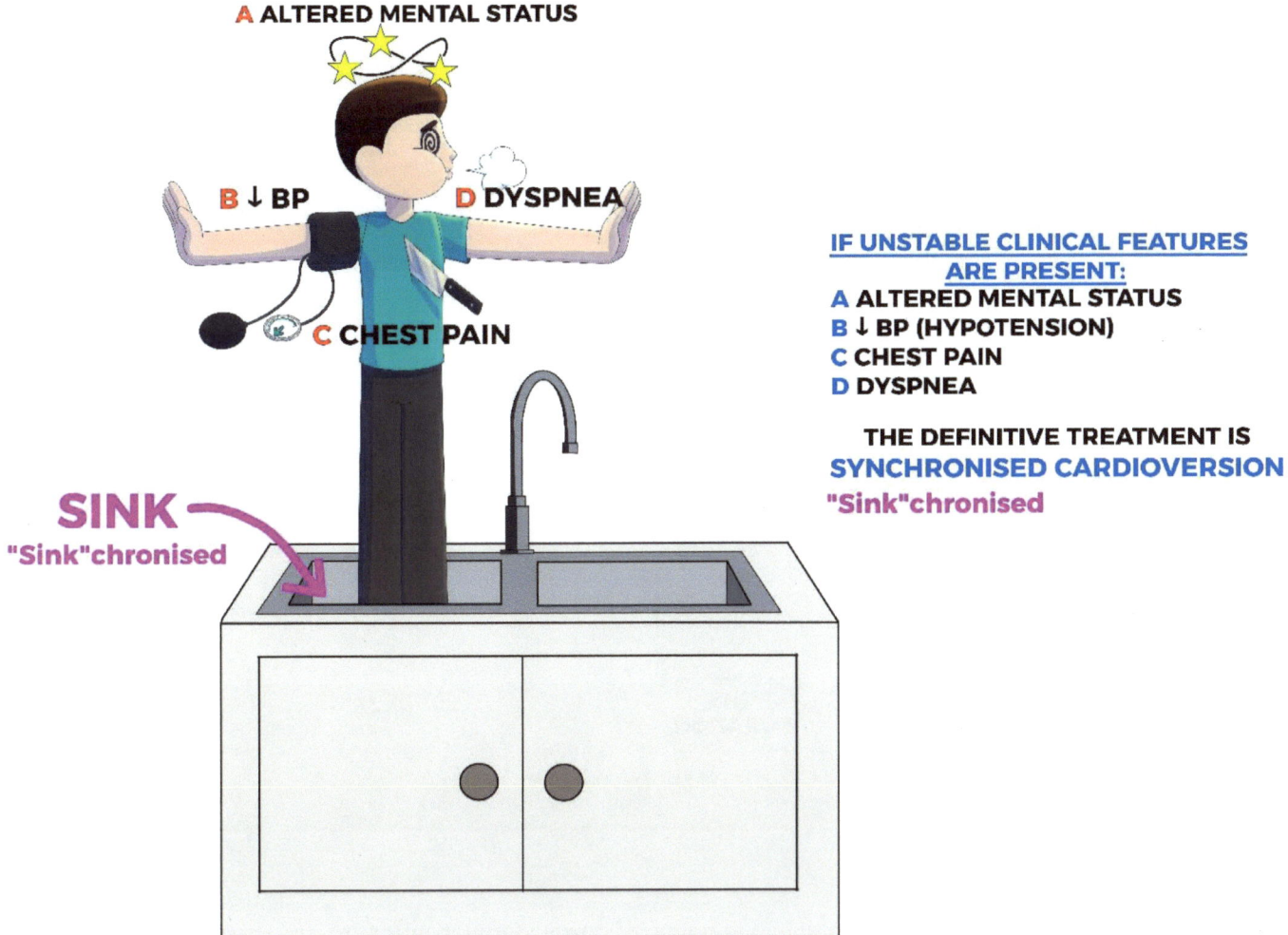

Medical students and doctors are often confused about which option to choose between synchronized cardioversion and unsynchronized cardioversion when answering a vignette with a patient with an arrhythmia with unstable clinical features. But after seeing this image, you will never forget that the treatment for a patient with an arrhythmia and **unstable symptoms** is **synchronized** ("Sink"chronised) **cardioversion** because this unstable patient is standing in a kitchen **SINK**.

Question 5:
A 57-year-old man is rushed to the ER after complaining of palpitations and shortness of breath. On examination, his blood pressure was 80/45 mmHg, and his respiratory rate was 22 breaths per minute. An EKG done shows Wolff Parkinson White Syndrome. What is the best treatment?
- A. Digoxin
- B. Procainamide
- C. Synchronized cardioversion
- D. Metoprolol

Question 5 answer: C. Synchronized cardioversion. Anytime you have an arrhythmia with unstable clinical features, the best treatment is synchronized cardioversion. Do not fall for the trap and pick the first-line treatment (in this case, procainamide). In this vignette, the unstable clinical features are hypotension (BP = 80/45mmHg) and shortness of breath with a respiratory rate of 22 breaths per minute.

CHAPTER 2:
EKG FOUNDATION

CARDIAC PHYSIOLOGY:

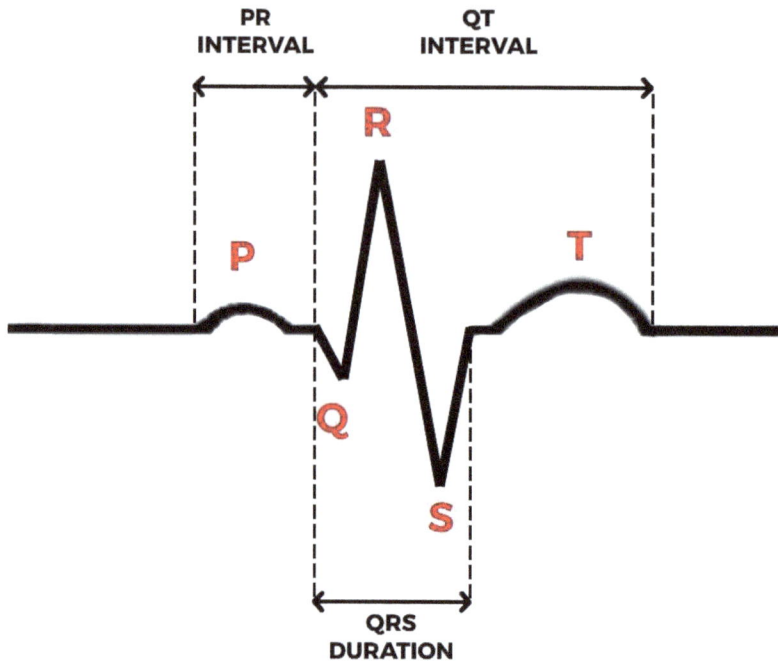

FIGURE 2 –2: PHYSIOLOGICAL PARTS OF THE CARDIAC CYCLE

P Wave: this represents atrial depolarization.

PR interval: this is the time duration from the beginning of atrial depolarization to the beginning of ventricular depolarization. It ranges from 120 – 200 ms (0.12 – 0.2 seconds).

QRS Complex: this represents ventricular depolarization. It ranges from 80 – 120 ms (0.08 – 0.12 seconds).

T wave: this represents ventricular repolarization.

QT interval: this is the time duration from ventricular contraction to ventricular relaxation. It ranges from 360 – 480 ms (0.36 – 0.48 seconds).

PACEMAKERS:

Typical pacemakers: These cells generate action potentials without an external stimulus. They stimulate the heart to beat in a normal, regular rhythm. Examples are the SA node, AV node, bundle of His, left and right bundle branches, and Purkinje fibers.

Ectopic pacemakers/ Automaticity foci: These cells generate action potentials without an external stimulus but make the heart beat abnormally outside of its normal rhythm. They cause some arrhythmias, such as atrial fibrillation, atrial flutter, ventricular fibrillation, ventricular tachycardia, premature atrial contraction, and premature ventricular contraction.

Artificial pacemakers: These are medical devices used to treat some arrhythmias. They generate action potentials that take over the activity of the SA node and regulate a patient's heart rate. There are two types: internal and external pacemakers.

CARDIAC ANATOMY:

Conduction system of the heart:
There are specialized cells in the heart called pacemakers. These cells generate action potentials that stimulate the heart muscles in the atria and ventricles to contract.
Impulses travel from the sinoatrial (SA) node to the atrioventricular (AV) node, then to the bundle of His, followed by the right and left bundle branches, and finally through the Purkinje fibers to reach the ventricles.

Pathway: SA node → AV node → Bundle of His → Right and Left bundle branch → Purkinje fibers → Ventricles.

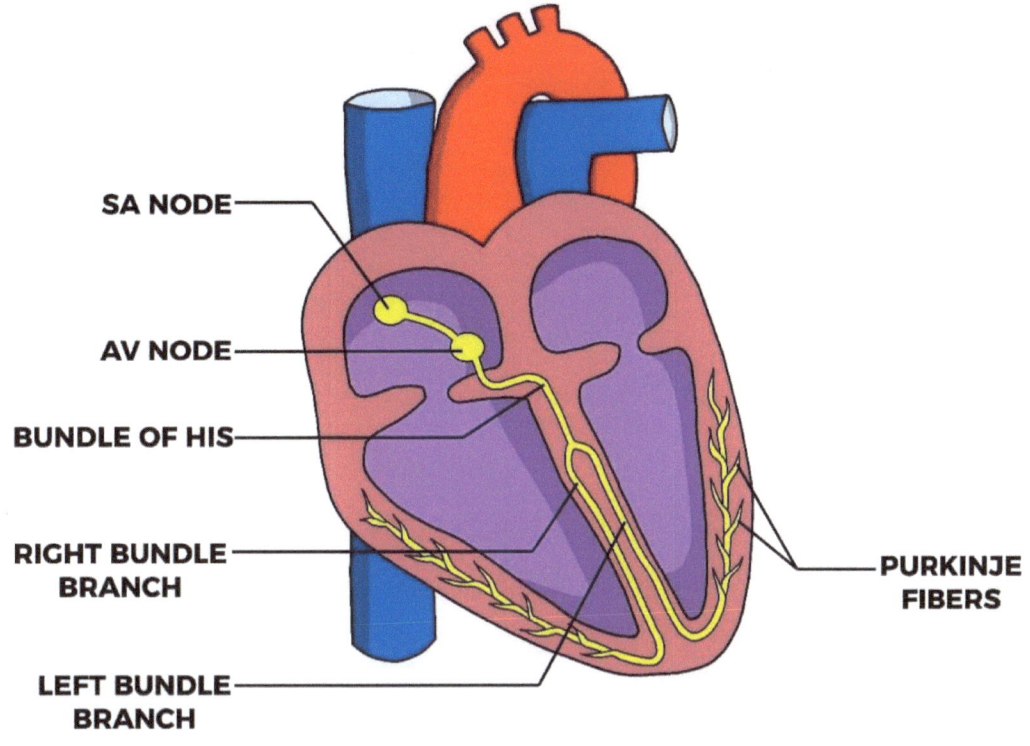

FIGURE 2 – 1: CONDUCTION SYSTEM OF THE HEART

Understanding the heart's conduction system is essential to comprehending the etiology of various arrhythmias. **Automaticity foci** are normal myocytes in the heart that become abnormal pacemaker cells. These abnormal pacemaker cells can now generate action potentials, stimulating the atria or ventricles to contract abnormally.
The following are the etiologies of the arrhythmias involving automaticity foci:

Atrial fibrillation:
This is caused by **multiple** automaticity foci in the **atrium**, which stimulate the atria to contract at a faster rate and **ir**regular rhythm.

Atrial flutter:
This is caused by a **single** automaticity focus in the **atrium**, which stimulates the atria to contract at a faster rate and **regular** rhythm.

Ventricular fibrillation:
This is caused by **multiple** automaticity foci in the **ventricle**, which stimulate the ventricles to contract at a faster rate and **ir**regular rhythm.

Ventricular tachycardia:
This is caused by a **single** automaticity focus in the **ventricle,** which stimulates the ventricles to contract at a faster rate and **regular** rhythm.

UNDERSTANDING THE EKG STRIP

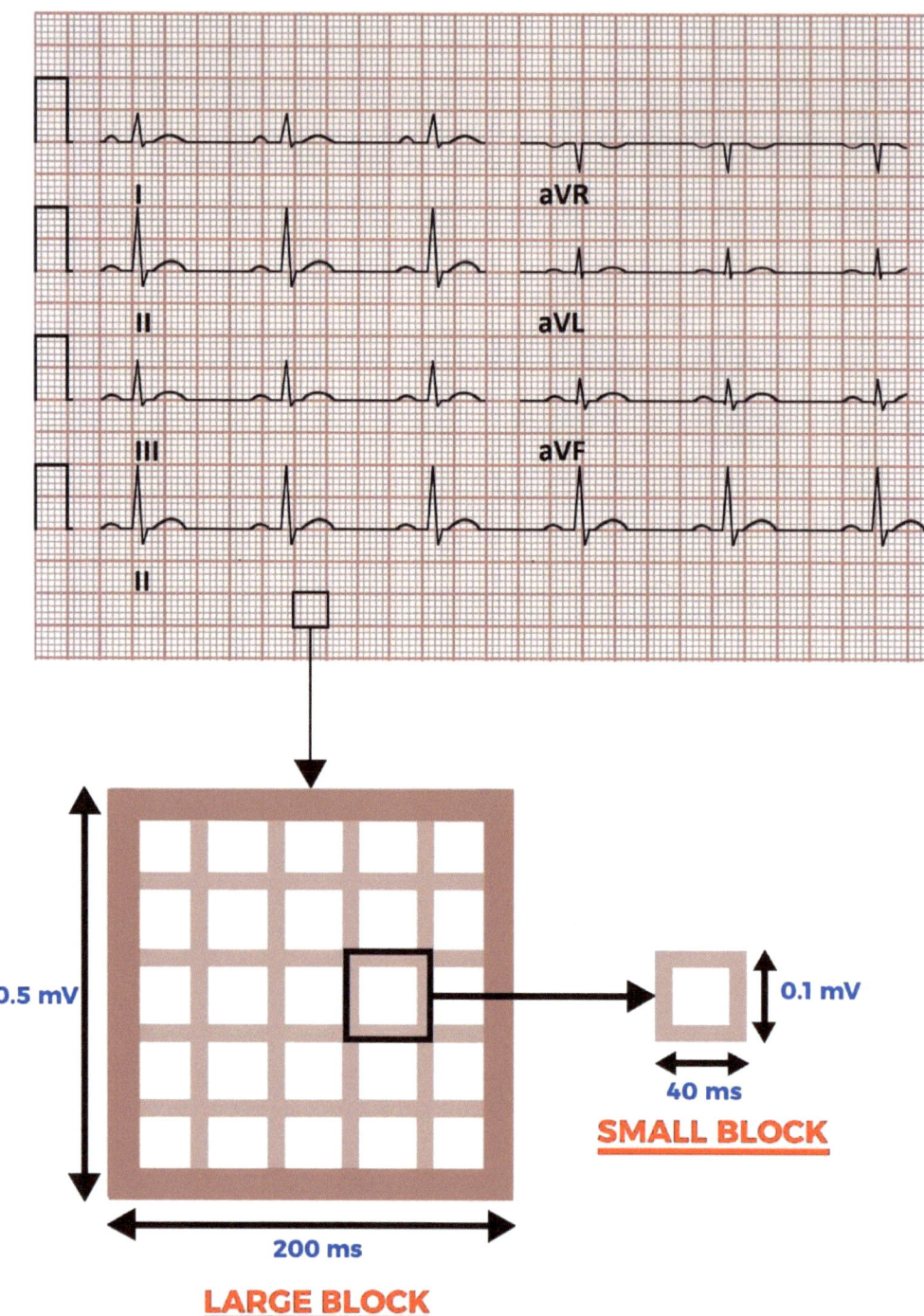

FIGURE 2 – 3: THE VALUES OF THE SMALL BLOCK AND LARGE BLOCK OF THE EKG

1 Small block horizontally = 40 ms (0.04 sec)

1 Small block vertically = 0.1 mV

1 Large block horizontally = 200 ms (0.2 sec)

1 Large block vertically = 0.5 mV

CAUSES OF CHANGES IN EKG INTERVALS AND DURATIONS:

PR interval: Normal range is **3 – 5** small blocks (120 – 200 ms or 0.12 – 0.2 seconds)

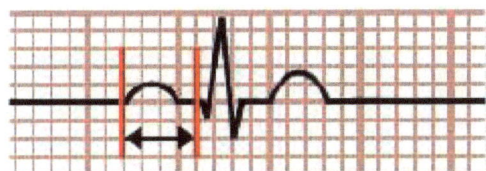

Causes of PR interval less than 120 ms (less than 3 small blocks)	Causes of PR interval greater than 200 ms (greater than 5 small blocks)
Wolff Parkinson white	First-degree heart block Second-degree heart block Third-degree heart block

QRS duration: Normal range is **2 – 3** small blocks (80 – 120 ms or 0.08 – 0.12 seconds)

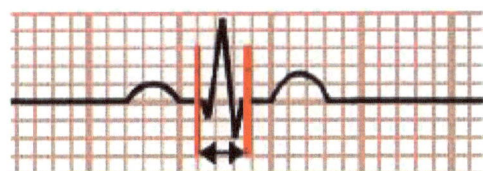

Causes of Narrow QRS duration less than 80 ms (less than 2 small blocks)	Causes of Wide QRS duration greater than 120 ms (greater than 3 small blocks)

Narrow QRS + Regular rhythm + Tachycardia
   A A Flutter (Narrow QRS)
   S SVT, ST (Narrow QRS)
	Wide QRS + Regular rhythm + Tachycardia
	   V V-Tach (Wide QRS)
	   W WPW (Wide QRS)

Narrow QRS + irregular rhythm + Tachycardia
   M MFAT (Narrow QRS)
   A A Fib (Narrow QRS)
	Wide QRS + irregular rhythm + Tachycardia
	   T Torsades de pointes (Wide QRS)
	   V V-Fib (Wide QRS)
	
	PVC (Premature ventricular contraction)

QT interval: Normal range is **8 – 12** small blocks (360 – 480 ms or 0.36 – 0.48 seconds)

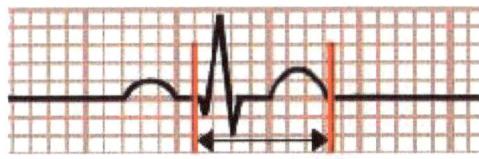

Causes of QT interval less than 360 ms	Causes of QT interval greater than 480 ms (greater than 2 large blocks + 2 small blocks)

Hypercalcemia	Hypocalcemia
	Congenital long QT syndrome:
	  1. Romano ward syndrome
	  2. Jervell and Lange Nielsen syndrome

V-Tach = Ventricular tachycardia; **V-Fib** = Ventricular Fibrillation; **WPW** = Wolff Parkinson White syndrome;
A Flutter = Atrial Flutter; **A Fib** = Atrial Fibrillation; **SVT** = Supraventricular Tachycardia; **ST** = Sinus tachycardia

CHAPTER 3:
UNDERSTANDING RATE AND RHYTHM

The two main characteristics of all arrhythmias are:

1. Rate
2. Rhythm

RATE:

The rate of each arrhythmia can be classified as follows:

1. Tachycardia: Rate is > 100 BPM
2. Normal rate: 60 – 100 BPM
3. Bradycardia: Rate is less than 60 BPM

A simple technique that can be used to estimate the heart rate on an EKG quickly:

The heart rate is greater than 100 BPM if the R waves are less than 3 large blocks apart.

Less than 3 Large blocks between two R waves = Heart rate is greater than 100 BPM (Tachycardia)

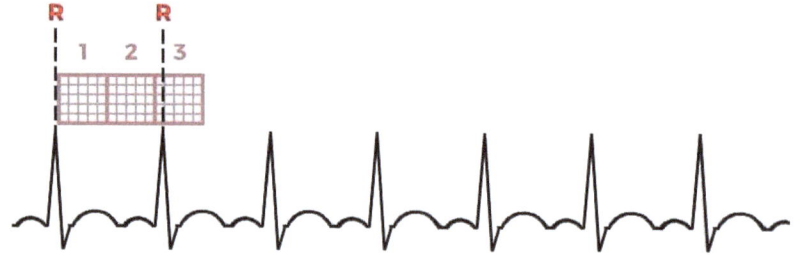

FIGURE 3 – 1: SIMPLE METHOD TO QUICKLY IDENTIFY TACHYCARDIA

The heart rate is less than 60 BPM if the R waves are greater than 5 large blocks apart.

Greater than 5 Large blocks between two R waves = Heart rate is less than 60 BPM (Bradycardia)

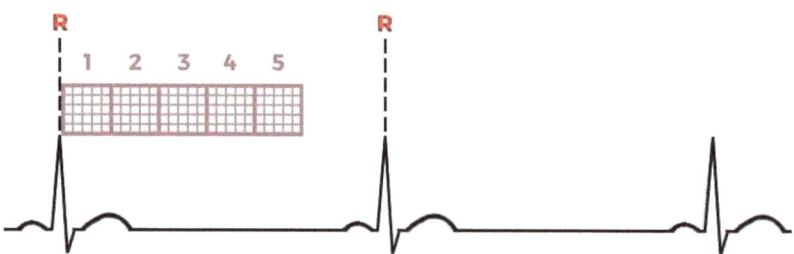

FIGURE 3 – 2: SIMPLE METHOD TO QUICKLY IDENTIFY BRADYCARDIA

R – R interval:

The R—R interval is the time duration between two successive R waves. The R wave is the R part of the Q "R" S (QRS) complex.

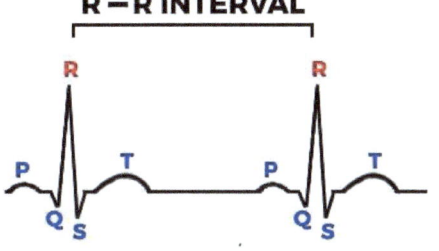

FIGURE 3 – 3: R – R INTERVAL

RHYTHMS:

The rhythm of each arrhythmia can be classified as follows:

1. Regular rhythm
2. Irregular rhythm

Regular rhythms:

All the R – R intervals are equal.

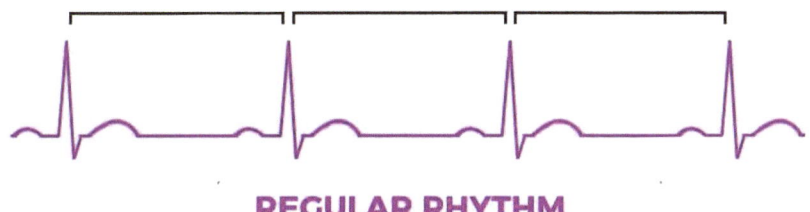

FIGURE 3 – 4: REGULAR RHYTHM WITH EQUAL R-R INTERVALS

Irregular rhythms:

All the R – R intervals are unequal.

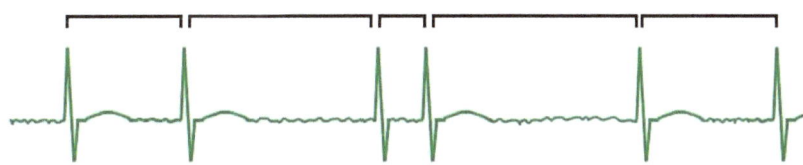

FIGURE 3 – 5: IRREGULAR RHYTHM WITH UNEQUAL R-R INTERVALS

CHAPTER 4:
THE FIVE STEPS USED TO INTERPRET ANY EKG

This quick five-step method is used to interpret any EKG in 10 seconds or less. These five steps involve identifying five characteristics of the arrhythmia on the EKG. These characteristics are:

RR PP QRS

1. **R** Rate
2. **R** Rhythm
3. **P** P wave
4. **P** PR interval
5. **QRS**

The mnemonic to remember these five characteristics is **RR PP QRS**. For any EKG question, always use this mnemonic to assess every EKG quickly. Sometimes, people rush and fail easy EKG questions by jumping to a wrong diagnosis just because they did not quickly asses these five characteristics. When looking at any EKG, always follow this sequence, and you will always have the required information to identify any arrhythmia. With practice, you will be able to assess these five characteristics in any EKG within a few seconds.

Because of how important these characteristics are, each arrhythmia in this book has been broken down into these five characteristics to enable you to identify each arrhythmia correctly and easily distinguish it from other arrhythmias.

Each of the five characteristics can have the following findings:

Rate: Bradycardia, normal rate or tachycardia
Rhythm: Regular or Irregular
P wave: Present, Absent or inverted. Check if all the P waves have the same shape. Also, check if all the P waves are related to the QRS or if the P waves are occurring independently of the QRS.
PR interval: Shortened, normal, or prolonged
QRS duration: Narrow, normal, or wide

The combination of findings of each of the five characteristics is unique to each arrhythmia.

For example:

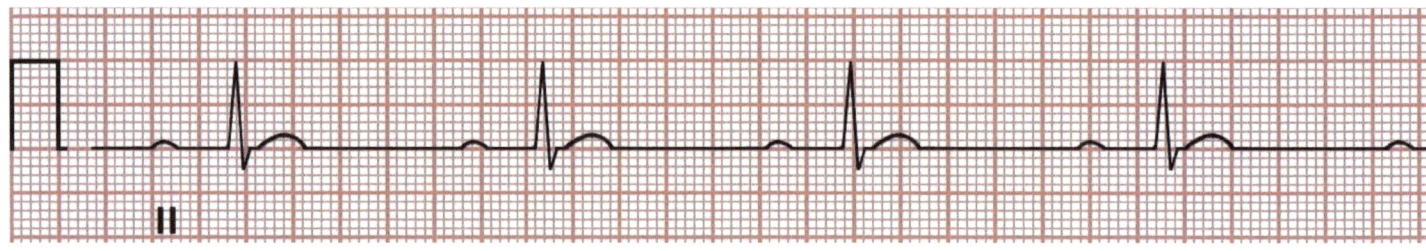

A patient with the combination of the following characteristics is classically seen in First-degree heart block:

Rate: Bradycardia (rate less than 60 BPM).
Rhythm: Regular P – P intervals and Regular R – R intervals.
P wave: Normal and present before every QRS
PR interval: Prolonged (>200 ms or 0.2 sec)
QRS duration: Normal

CHAPTER 5:
ARRHYTHMIAS

Since we have understood the difference between regular and irregular rhythms and narrow and wide QRS durations, we can now classify all the arrhythmias. By learning how to classify all arrhythmias, you will be able to diagnose any arrhythmia in any EKG question and rule out other wrong options. Learning this classification is very high yield.

CLASSIFICATION OF ARRHYTHMIAS:

TACHYCARDIA (> 100 BPM)	BRADYCARDIA (LESS THAN 50 BPM)	NORMAL RATE: 60 – 100 BPM

Regular rhythm: V WAS
V V-Tach (Wide QRS)
W WPW (Wide QRS)
A A Flutter (Narrow QRS)
S SVT, ST (Narrow QRS)
 	
Irregular rhythm: TVMA
T Torsades de pointes (Wide QRS)
V V-Fib (Wide QRS)
M MFAT (Narrow QRS)
A A Fib (Narrow QRS)
	Bradycardia + Regular rhythm + Normal PR interval:
	Sinus bradycardia
	
	Bradycardia + Regular rhythm + Increased PR interval:
	First-degree Heart block
	Third-degree heart block
	
	Bradycardia + irregular rhythm + Increased PR interval:
	Second-degree type 1
	Second-degree type 2
		Regular rhythm:
		Sinus rhythm
		First-degree Heart block
		
		Irregular rhythm:
		Wandering pacemaker
		
		Ectopic beats:
		Premature Atrial Contraction (PAC)
		Premature Ventricular contraction (PVC)
		
		Other EKG Findings: CHAPS
		C Congenital long QT syndrome:
		  1. Romano ward syndrome
		  2. Jervell and Lange Nielsen syndrome
		
		H Hypothermia: Osborne wave
		
		H Hypo/ Hyper: Calcium, Potassium
		
		A Asystole
		
		P Pulseless electrical activity
		
		P Pericardial effusion electrical alternans
		
		P Pulmonary embolism
		
		S ST elevation/ Depression:

V-Tach = Ventricular tachycardia; **V-Fib** = Ventricular Fibrillation; **WPW** = Wolff Parkinson White syndrome;
A Flutter = Atrial Flutter; **A Fib** = Atrial Fibrillation; **SVT** = Supraventricular Tachycardia; **ST** = Sinus tachycardia

Tachycardia + Regular Arrhythmias:

VENTRICULAR TACHYCARDIA

Single EKG strip:

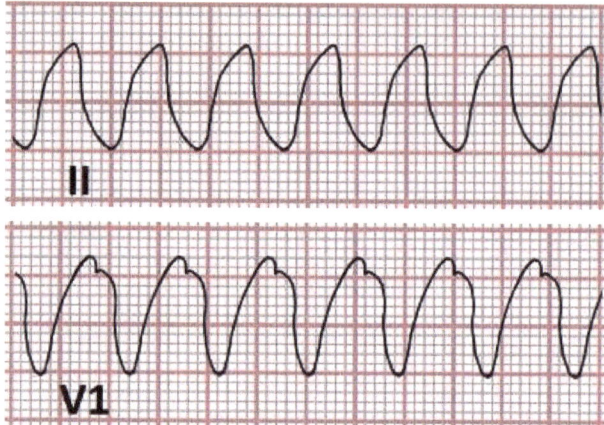

FIGURE 5 – 1: VENTRICULAR TACHYCARDIA

Etiology:
This is caused by a single automaticity focus in the ventricle, which stimulates the ventricles to contract at a faster rate and regular rhythm. Here, the automaticity focus stimulates the ventricle to contract regularly (unlike Ventricular fibrillation, which has a regular rhythm). Sustained ventricular tachycardia is life-threatening because the ventricular contractions it produces are rapid but weak. These weak ventricular contractions are not strong enough to push an adequate amount of blood out of the ventricles. As a result, there is very low or no cardiac output, leading to the cessation of blood circulation. The lack of blood circulation causes pulselessness, low blood pressure, and loss of consciousness.

Causes: (HEAT DRUGS):
H Heart disorders like cardiomyopathy, aortic stenosis
E Electrolyte disorders: Hypokalemia, hypomagnesemia
A Acute myocardial infarction (especially within the first 24 hr.).
T Torsades de pointes
Drugs that prolong QT interval: **ABCDE**
    Anti-**A**rrhythmia class **1**A, **3** (13 Friday the 13th)
    Anti-**B**iotic: Macrolide: Azithromycin, Clarithromycin, and Erythromycin
    Anti-Psy**C**hotic: Haloperidol
    Anti-**D**epressant: Tricyclic Antidepressant (TCA)
    Anti-**E**metic: Ondansetron

EKG findings:
Rate: Tachycardia
Rhythm: Regular
P wave: None
PR interval: None
QRS: Wide (greater than 120 ms)

Clinical Features: PUB
P Pulseless
U Unconscious
B BP Low (Hypotensive)

Treatment:
Follow the ACLS flow chart

ACLS flow chart:

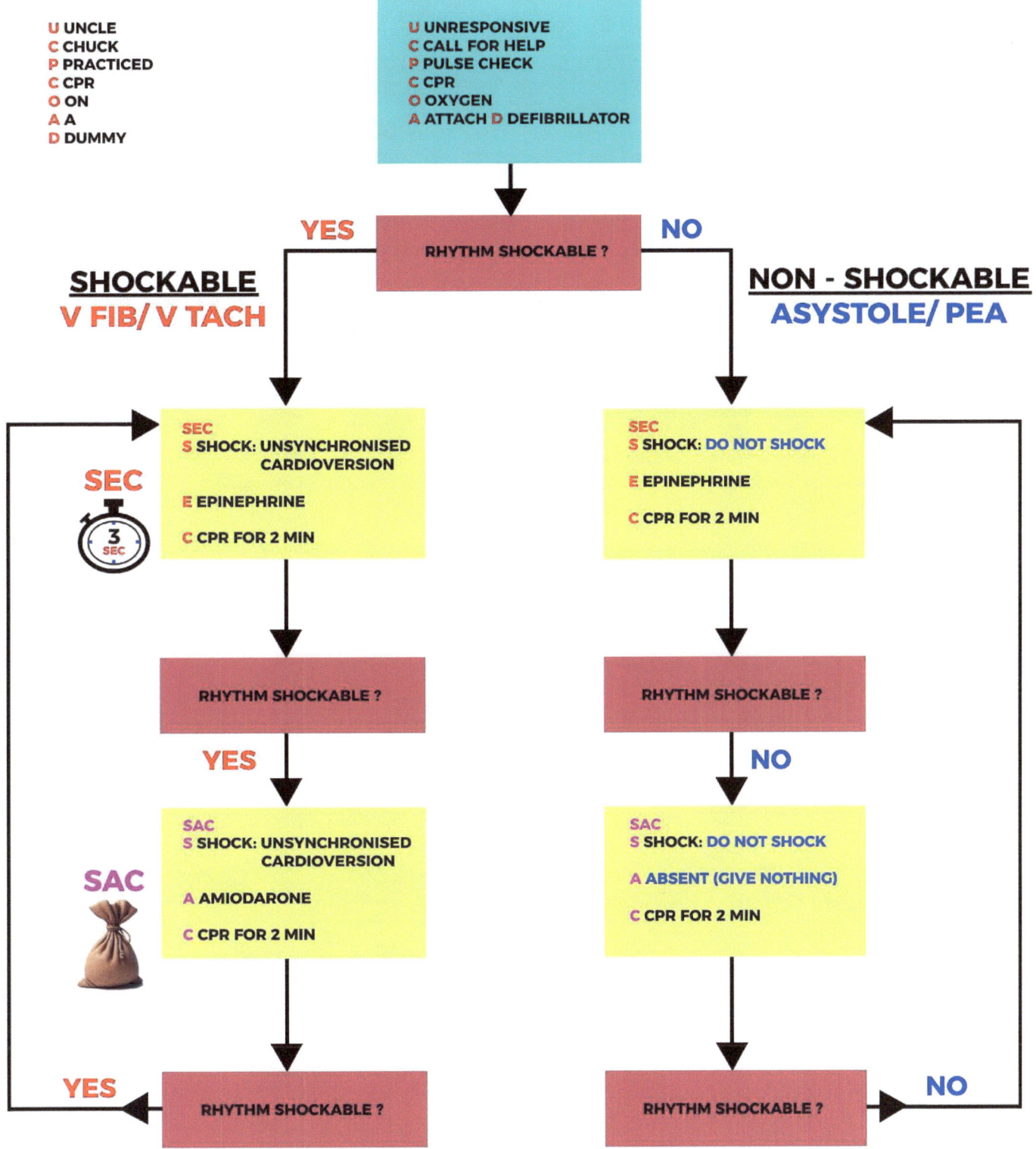

FIGURE 5 – 2: ACLS TREATMENT FLOWCHART FOR VENTRICULAR TACHYCARDIA

FIGURE 5 – 3: VENTRICULAR TACHYCARDIA

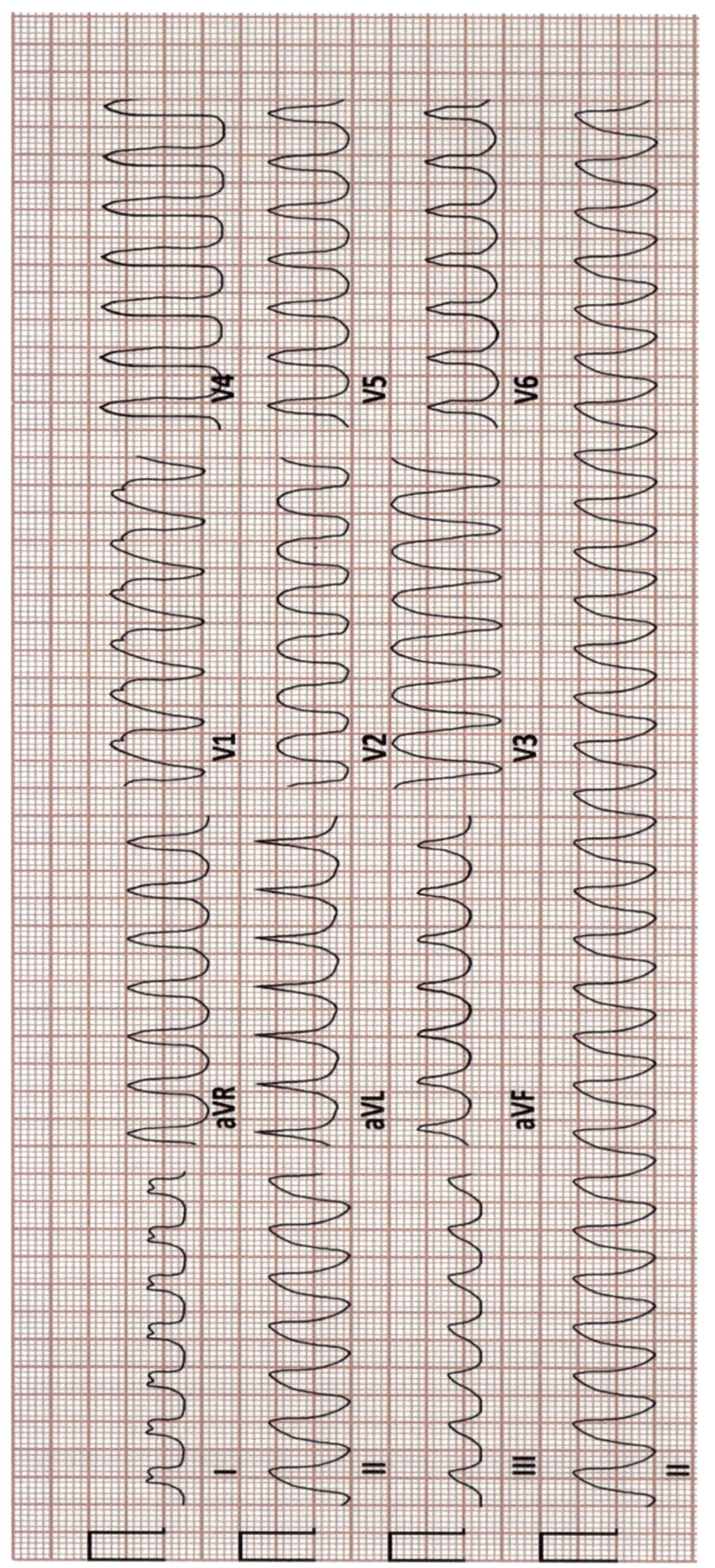

EKG findings:
Rate: Tachycardia
Rhythm: Regular
P wave: None
PR interval: None
QRS: Wide (greater than 120 ms)

Question 6:
A 62-year-old man under admission suddenly lost consciousness while talking to you. He was receiving treatment for congestive heart failure and uncontrolled vomiting. He has been receiving his regular heart failure medications and Ondansetron for vomiting. On examination, he was unconscious and unarousable, pulseless, and his blood pressure was 30/10 mmHg. What is the next best step?
   A. Synchronized cardioversion
   B. Call for help
   C. Oxygen
   D. Start CPR

Question 6 answer: B. Call for help.
This question is focused on assessing your ability to manage a hypotensive and unconscious patient that requires you to follow the ACLS flow chart. You can remember the first steps in the ACLS flow chart by remembering this mnemonic:
UCPCOAD: U Uncle, C Chuck, P Practices, C CPR, O On, A A, D Dummy.
UCPCOAD: This stands for:
U Unconscious.
C Call for help
P Pulse rate
C CPR
O Oxygen
A Attach
D Defibrillator

This is a trick question that most people overlook and fail. Always remember to call for help first before starting CPR.

WOLFF PARKINSON WHITE SYNDROME (WPW)

Single EKG strip:

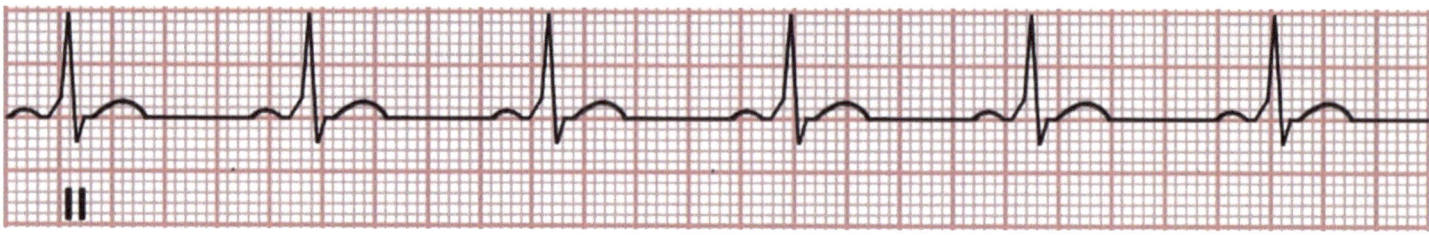

FIGURE 5 – 4: WOLFF PARKINSON WHITE SYNDROME

Diagram:

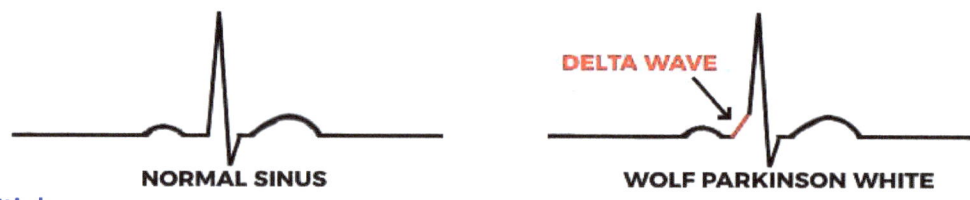

Etiology:
This is due to the presence of an abnormal connection between the atria and ventricles by an accessory pathway. This accessory pathway is called the bundle of Kent. Normally, the action potential produced by the SA node passes through the AV node before it reaches the ventricles. However, in WPW, the action potential produced by the SA node bypasses the AV node and moves in a forward direction (**anterograde**) through the bundle of Kent to the ventricles, causing an **early** depolarization of a portion of the ventricle, resulting in the formation of the Delta wave. The Delta wave causes the QRS duration to be longer than normal. The bundle of Kent also creates a unique type of tachycardia called **Atrioventricular Re-entrant Tachycardia (AVRT)**. In AVRT, the action potential produced by the SA node, which reaches the ventricles, leaves the ventricles in a backward direction (**retrograde**) through the bundle of Kent and quickly restimulates the atria, eventually resulting in tachycardia.
(Note: Atrioventricular nodal re-entrant tachycardia (AVNRT) occurs in supraventricular tachycardia)

EKG Findings:
Rate: Tachycardia
Rhythm: Regular
P wave: Normal
PR interval: Shortened (less than 120 ms)
QRS: Wide (greater than 120 ms)
+
Delta wave (slow upstroke of the initial portion of QRS)

Clinical Features:
Caucasian man
Tall
+
P Palpitation
P Pulse: Tachycardia and Regular

Lab:
Best initial test: EKG

Treatment:
1st line treatment: Procainamide
(Avoid Calcium channel blockers (CCB) or Digoxin because these drugs block the passage of impulses through the normal conduction pathway and increase the passage of impulses through the bundle of Kent)

FIGURE 5 – 5: WOLFF PARKINSON WHITE SYNDROME

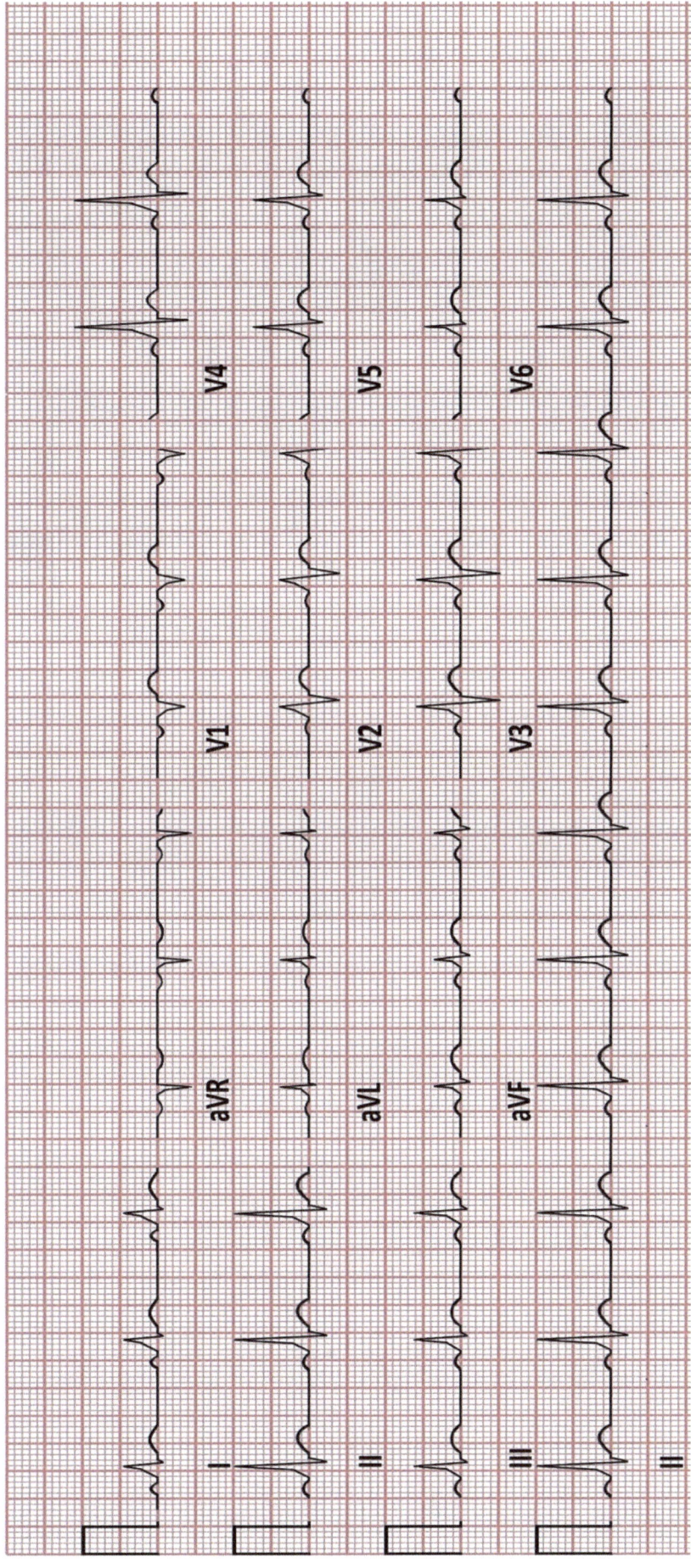

EKG Findings:
Rate: Tachycardia
Rhythm: Regular
P wave: Normal
PR interval: Shortened (less than 120 ms)
QRS: Wide (greater than 120 ms)
+
Delta wave (slow upstroke of the initial portion of QRS)

ATRIAL FLUTTER

Single EKG strip

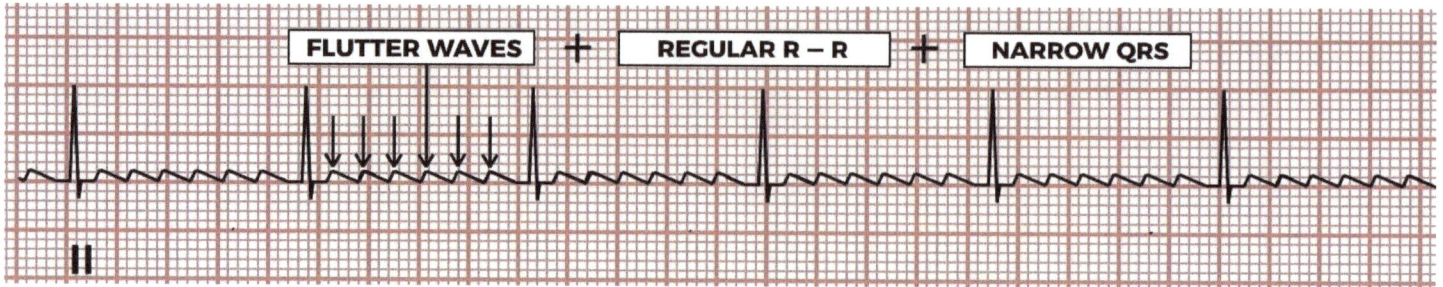

FIGURE 5 – 6: ATRIAL FLUTTER

Etiology:
This is caused by a single automaticity focus in the atrium, which stimulates the atria to contract at a faster rate and regular rhythm. Here, the automaticity focus stimulates the atria to contract regularly (unlike atrial fibrillation, which has an irregular rhythm). These regular contractions produce flutter waves that are identical in height and width.

Causes:
Hyperthyroidism

EKG Findings:
Rate: Tachycardia
Rhythm: Regular R-R intervals
P wave: None
PR interval: None
QRS: Narrow (less than 80 ms)
+
Flutter waves: All flutter waves are identical, have the same height and width, and are equally spaced.
(Note: Fibrillary waves seen in atrial fibrillation are not identical and have unequal height and width).

Clinical Features:
Asymptomatic: Most patients are asymptomatic
OR
Symptomatic
Fatigue
Lightheadedness
P Palpitation
P Pulse: Tachycardia and regular

Lab:
Best initial test: EKG
Transthoracic Echocardiography
CMP
CBC
Thyroid function test

Treatment:

If moderate or severe mitral valve disease is present:
A Anticoagulant: Warfarin MUST be used if moderate or severe mitral valve disease is present
R Rate control: Both Calcium Channel Blockers: Diltiazem, or Beta Blocker: Metoprolol are **1st line**
R Rhythm control: Amiodarone

No mitral valve disease:
A Anticoagulant: Aspirin, Novel anticoagulant (NAC), or Warfarin (depending on the CHADS Score)
   a. CHADS Score of 0 = No Anticoagulant required

   b. CHADS Score of 1 = Give Aspirin, Warfarin or Novel anticoagulant: Dabigatran, Rivaroxaban, Apixaban

   c. CHADS Score of ≥ 2 = Give Warfarin or Novel anticoagulant: Dabigatran, Rivaroxaban, Apixaban (Never give Aspirin when the CHAD Score is equal to or greater than 2)

R Rate control: Both Calcium Channel Blockers: Diltiazem, or Beta Blocker: Metoprolol are **1st line**
R Rhythm control: Amiodarone

CHADS Score:
The whole point of calculating the CHADS score is that the number you obtain at the end of the calculation will be used to select an anticoagulant to be given to the patient with Atrial Flutter.

CHADS VAS

CRITERIA	POINTS
C CHF	1
H HTN	1
A Age > 75 *	1
A Age > 75 *	1
D DM	1
S Stroke/ TIA	1
S Stroke/ TIA	1
V Vascular disease: CAD	1
A Age 65 – 75 *	1
S Sex: Female	1
TOTAL	9

CHF = Congestive Heart failure; **HTN** = Hypertension;
DM = Diabetes Mellitus; **TIA** = Transient Ischemic Attack; **CAD** = Coronary Artery Disease.
* = If the patient's age is between 65 – 75 years, they score 1 point, but if the patients age is > 75 years they score 2 points.

FIGURE 5 – 7: ATRIAL FLUTTER

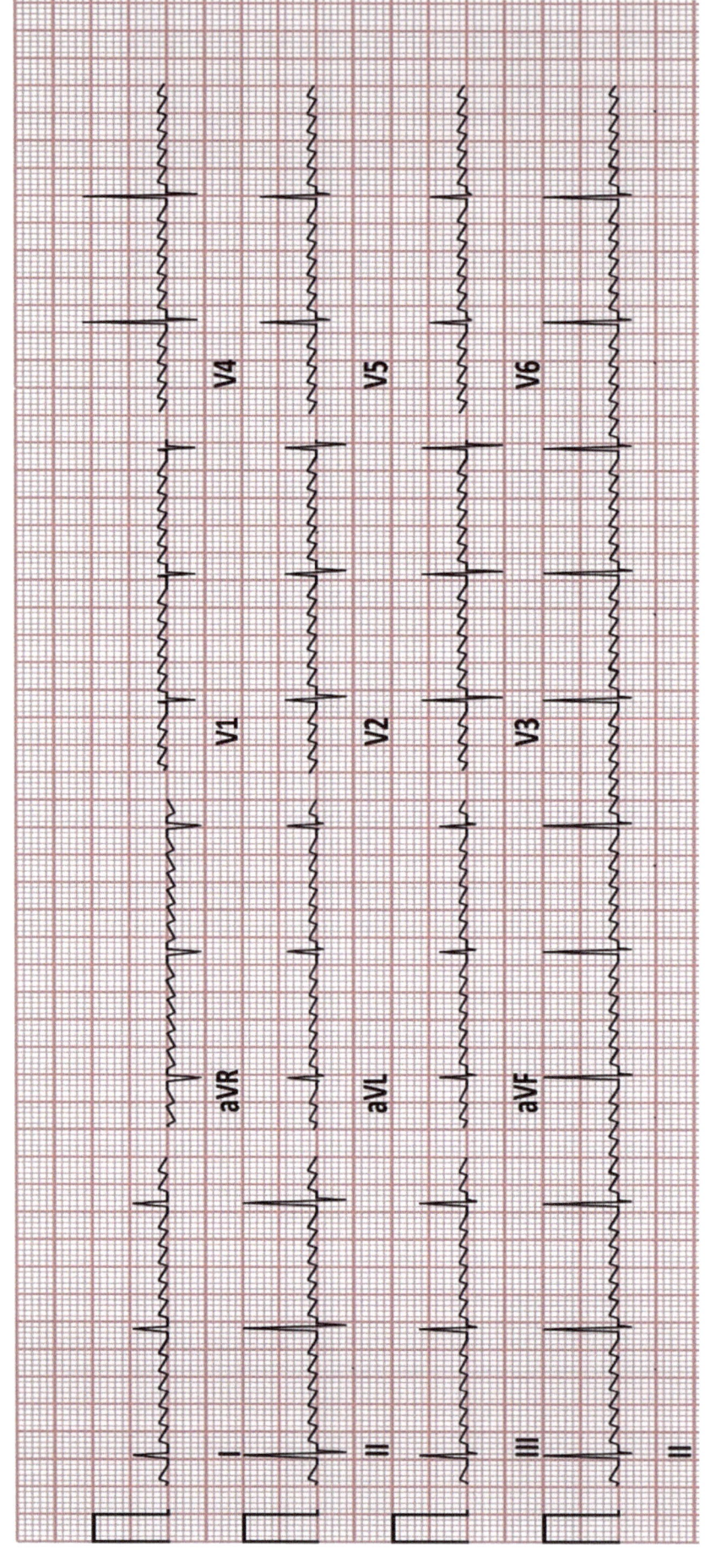

EKG Findings:
Rate: Tachycardia
Rhythm: Regular R-R intervals
P wave: None
PR interval: None
QRS: Narrow (less than 80 ms)
+
Flutter waves: All flutter waves are identical, have the same height and width, and are equally spaced.

Question 7:
An 82-year-old female comes to the ER complaining of dizziness and palpitations. She has had a history of diabetes mellitus and hypertension for 45 years and is compliant with all her medication. Her BMI is 39, and she has smoked a pack of cigarettes daily for 34 years. On examination, her pulse is regular. An EKG shows Atrial Flutter. What is the etiology of atrial flutter?
  A. Multiple automaticity foci in the ventricle
  B. Bundle of Kent
  C. Single automaticity focus in the atrium
  D. Atrial muscle scaring

Question 7: The answer is C. Atrial flutter is caused by a single automaticity focus in the atrium, which stimulates the atria to contract at a faster rate and regular rhythm.

Question 8:
An 82-year-old female comes to the ER complaining of dizziness and palpitations. She has had a history of diabetes mellitus and hypertension for 45 years and is compliant with all her medication. Her BMI is 39, and she has smoked a pack of cigarettes daily for 34 years. On examination, her pulse is regular. The EKG done is shown below. What is the best treatment?

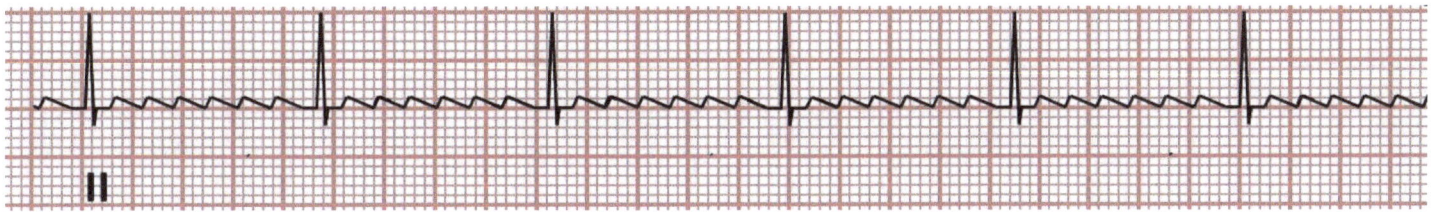

  A. Aspirin
  B. Warfarin

Question 8: The answer is B, Warfarin. For this question, you first have to calculate the CHADS Score:
1. Hypertension: 1
2. Diabetes Mellitus: 1
3. Age > 75: 1
4. Age > 75: 1
5. Female: 1
The CHADS Score for this patient = 5

CHADS Score of ≥ 2 = Give Warfarin or Novel anticoagulant: Dabigatran, Rivaroxaban, Apixaban (Never give Aspirin when the CHAD Score is equal to or greater than 2)

SINUS TACHYCARDIA

Single EKG strip

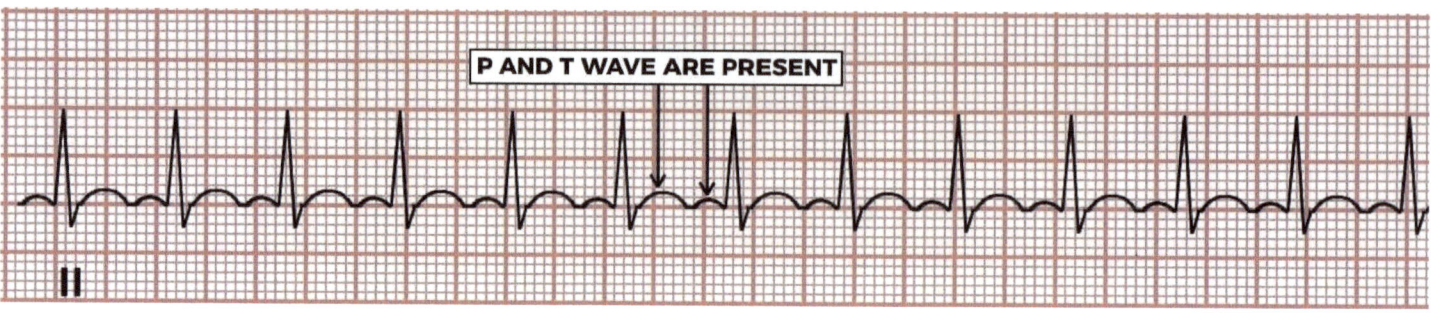

FIGURE 5 – 8: SINUS TACHYCARDIA

Etiology:
This occurs when the SA node stimulates the heart to beat faster than 100 beats per minute. The causes of sinus tachycardia may be physiologic or pathologic.

Causes:
1. Physiologic PEA
P Pain
E Exercise
A Anxiety

2. Pathologic
Hyperthyroidism
Anemia
Fever

EKG findings:
Rate: Tachycardia
Rhythm: Regular
P wave: Normal and P wave is always present
PR interval: Normal
QRS: Narrow (less than 80 ms)

To differentiate sinus tachycardia (ST) from supraventricular tachycardia (SVT), sinus tachycardia has both P and T waves present. In supraventricular tachycardia, the P wave is usually buried within the T wave, making only the T wave visible.

Clinical Features:
P Palpitation
P Pulse: Tachycardia and regular

Lab:
Best initial test: EKG

Treatment:
1. Physiologic sinus tachycardia: Reassure only

2. Pathologic sinus tachycardia: Treat the underlying cause

FIGURE 5 – 9: SINUS TACHYCARDIA

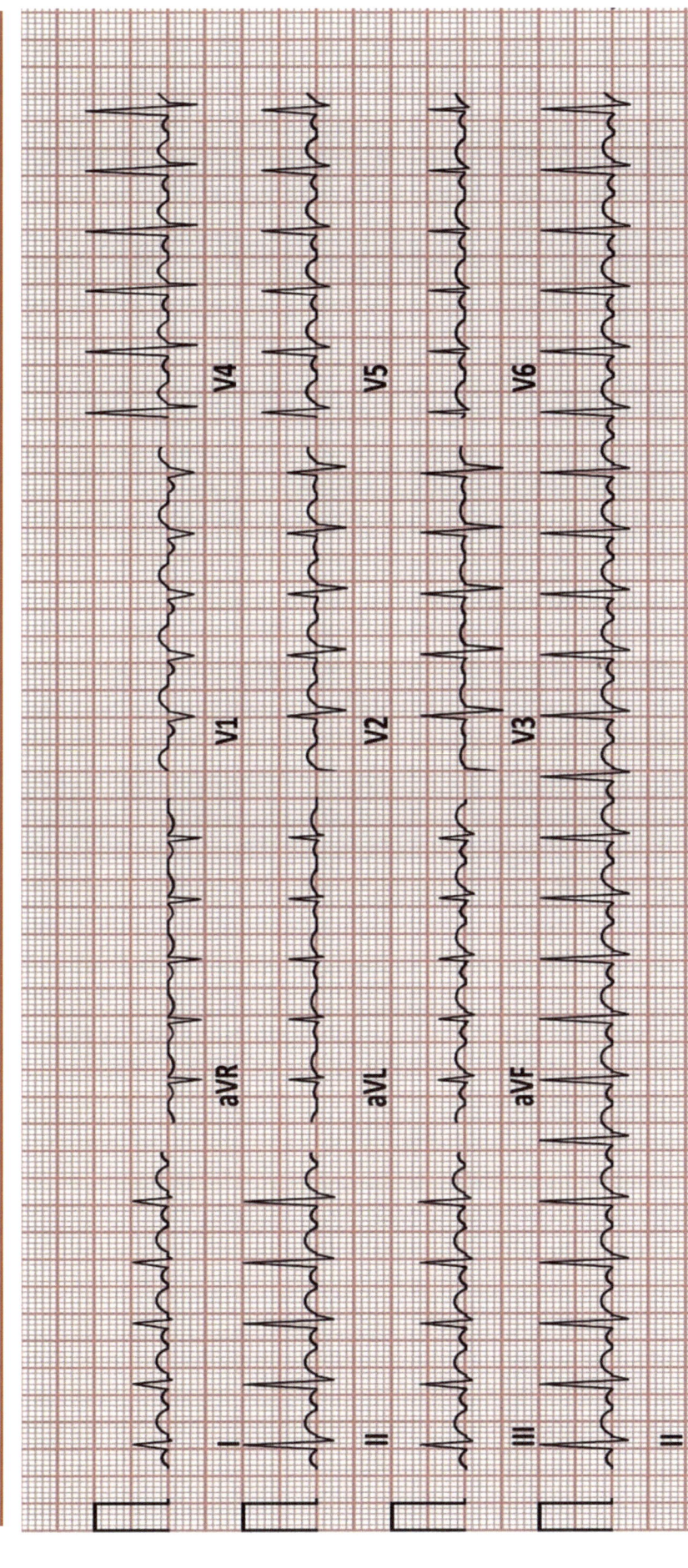

EKG findings:
Rate: Tachycardia
Rhythm: Regular
P wave: Normal and P wave is always present
PR interval: Normal
QRS: Narrow (less than 80 ms)

SUPRAVENTRICULAR TACHYCARDIA

Single EKG strip

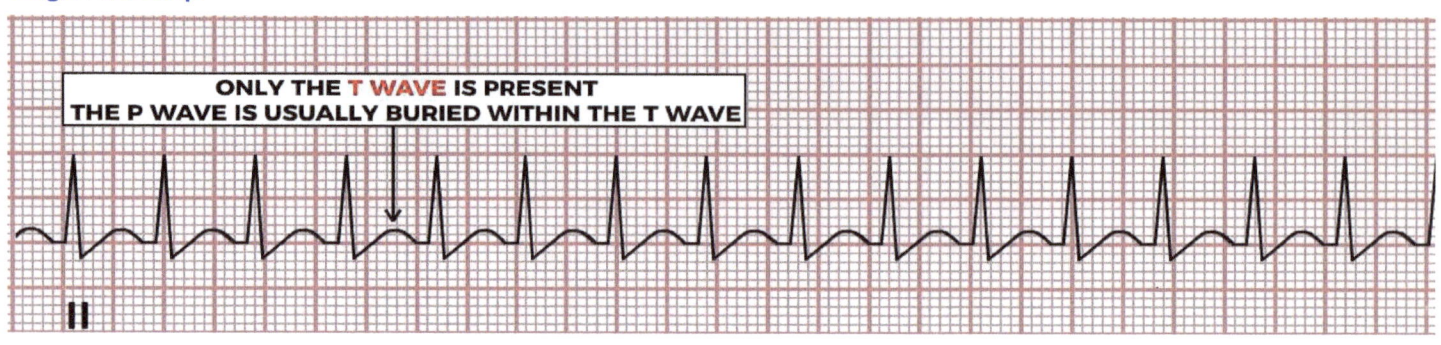

FIGURE 5 – 10: SUPRAVENTRICULAR TACHYCARDIA

Etiology:

Supraventricular tachycardia (SVT) is a term used to describe multiple tachycardias originating above the ventricle. SVT can be caused by atrioventricular nodal re-entrant tachycardia (AVnRT). This is due to a re-entry circuit involving the AV node. An atrial ectopic beat occurring at precisely the right time will create a re-entry circuit continuously through the AV node that will simultaneously rapidly stimulate the atria and the ventricles, causing tachycardia. It can also be due to a congenital structural defect in the bundle of His.
(Note: A similar type of tachycardia (without "Nodal" in the name) called AVRT Atrioventricular Re- entrant tachycardia (AVRT) is seen in Wolff Parkinson white syndrome)

EKG findings:
Rate: Tachycardia, usually greater than 150 BPM
Rhythm: Regular
P wave: The P wave is usually not visible because it is buried within the T wave. This happens because the rate is too rapid.
PR interval: Usually not measurable
QRS: Narrow (less than 80 ms)

Clinical Features:
P Pulse: Tachycardia and regular
P Palpitation

Lab:
Best initial test: EKG

Treatment:
Best initial treatment: Vasovagal maneuver
↓
Next best treatment: IV Adenosine

Prevention of reoccurrence:
Either Calcium Channel Blocker: Diltiazem or Beta Blocker: Metoprolol

---

Vasovagal maneuvers:
Pathophysiology:
Vasovagal maneuvers increase parasympathetic activity, causing a decrease in the heart rate.

Examples: ABCDE Squatting
A V**A**lsalva maneuver (exhalation against a closed airway)
B Breath holding
C Carotid sinus massage
D Dipping face in cold water
E Eye ball pressure
Squatting

FIGURE 5 – 11: SUPRAVENTRICULAR TACHYCARDIA

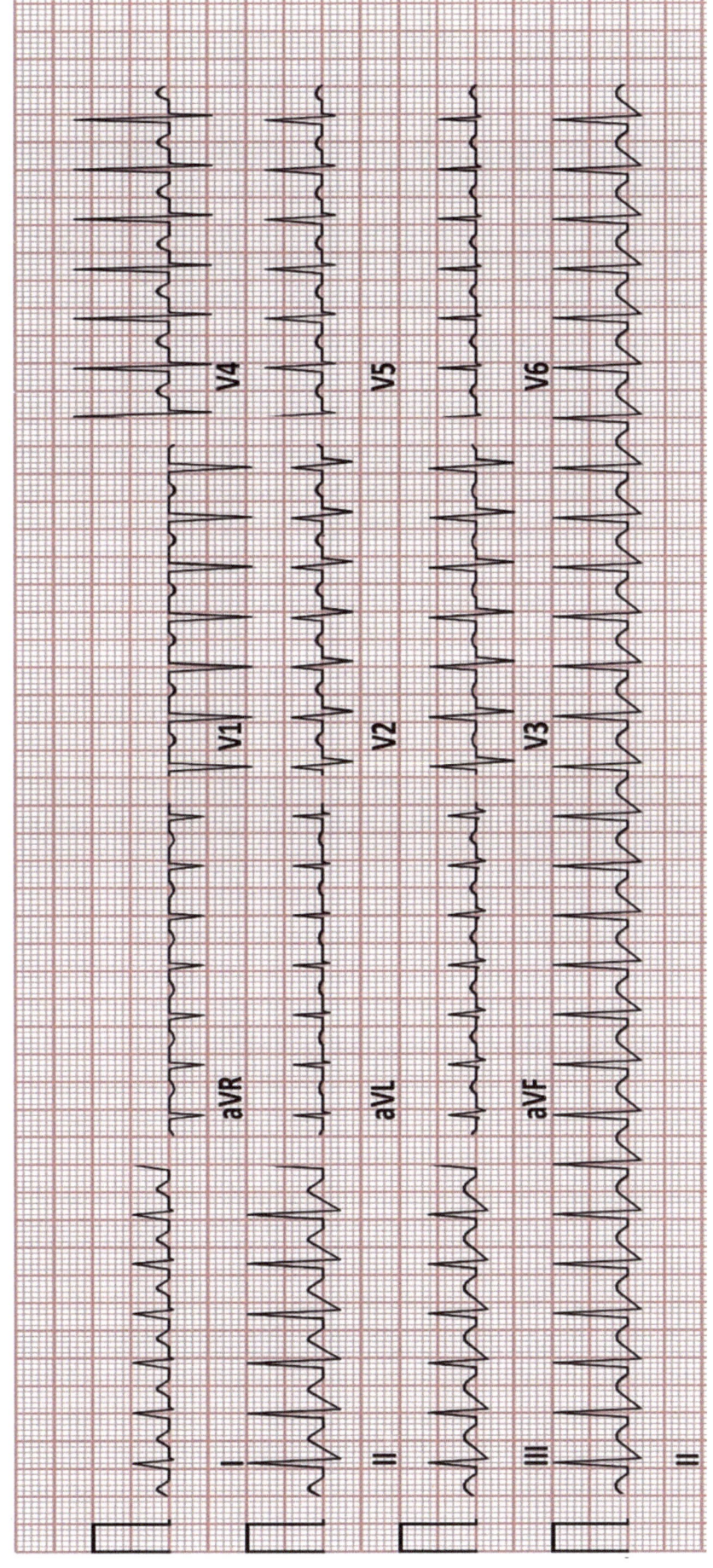

EKG findings:
Rate: Tachycardia, usually greater than 150 BPM
Rhythm: Regular
P wave: The P wave is usually buried within the T wave because the rate is too rapid.
PR interval: Usually not measurable
QRS: Narrow (less than 80 ms)

Tachycardia + Irregular Arrhythmias:

TORSADES DE POINTES

Single EKG strip

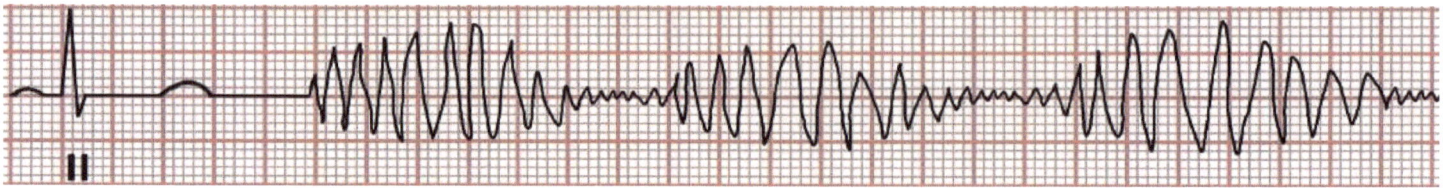

FIGURE 5 – 12: TORSADES DE POINTES

Etiology:
Torsades de pointes is caused by anything that can prolong the QT interval.

Causes:
Two main things that increase the QT intervals are:

1. Congenital long QT syndrome:
Roman ward
Jervell and Lange Nielsen

2. Drugs: ABCDE
Anti-**A**rrhythmia class **1**A, **3** (13 Friday the 13th)
Anti-**B**iotic: Macrolide: Azithromycin, Clarithromycin and Erythromycin
Anti-Psy**C**hotic: Haloperidol
Anti-**D**epressant: Tricyclic Antidepressant (TCA)
Anti-**E**metic: Ondansetron

EKG
Rate: Tachycardia
Rhythm: Irregular
P wave: Absent
PR interval: None
QRS: Wide (greater than 120 ms)
QT interval: Prolonged QT interval preceding the torsade's de pointe
The EKG is described as the QRS complexes twisting along the isoelectric line, with an increase and decrease in the amplitude of the QRS.

Clinical Features:
History of ingestion of drugs that prolong the QT interval
+
P Pulse: Tachycardia and irregular
P Palpitation

Lab:
Best initial test: EKG

Treatment:
IV Magnesium Sulfate

To prevent further episodes:
Beta Blockers

FIGURE 5 – 13: TORSADES DE POINTES

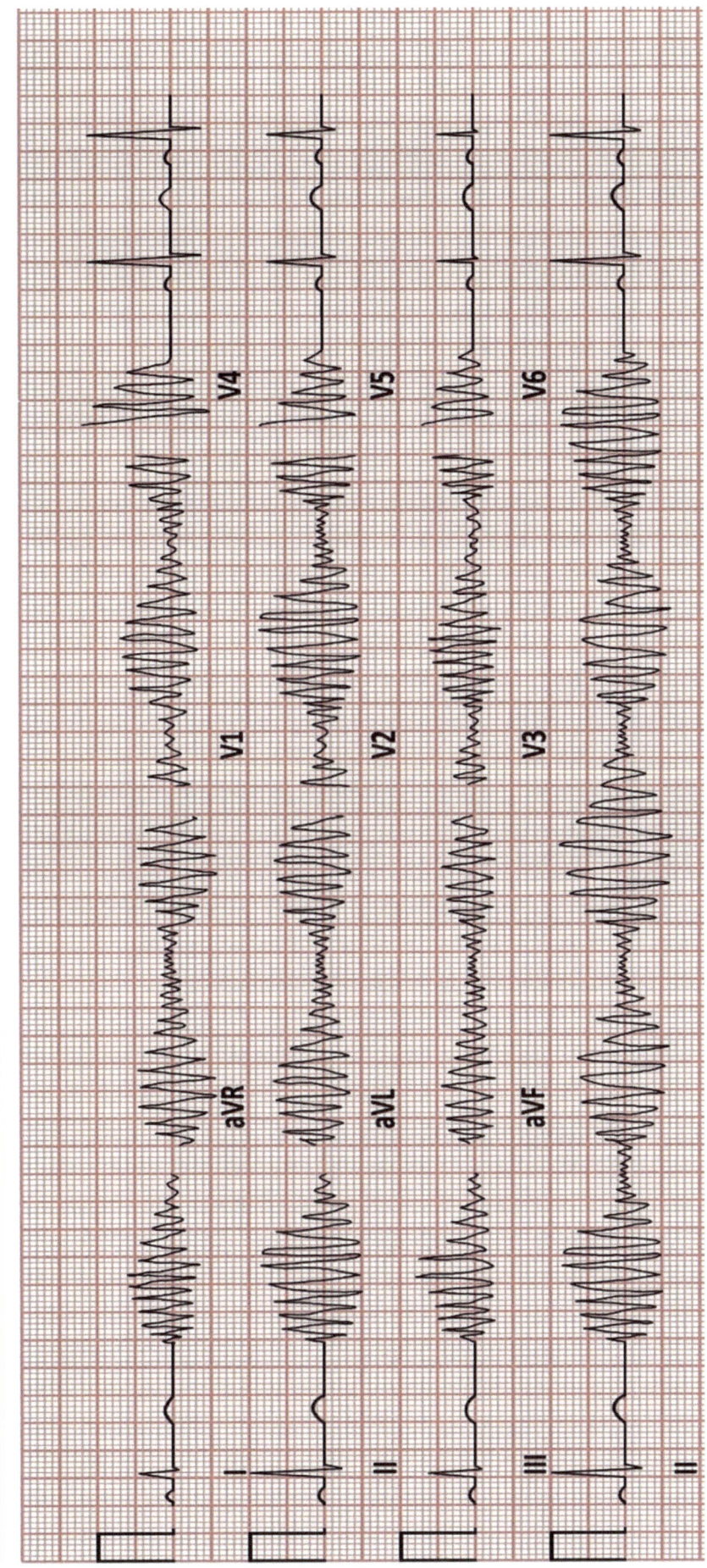

EKG
Rate: Tachycardia
Rhythm: Irregular
P wave: Absent
PR interval: None
QRS: Wide (greater than 120 ms)
QT interval: Prolonged QT interval preceding the torsade's de pointe

VENTRICULAR FIBRILLATION

Single EKG strip

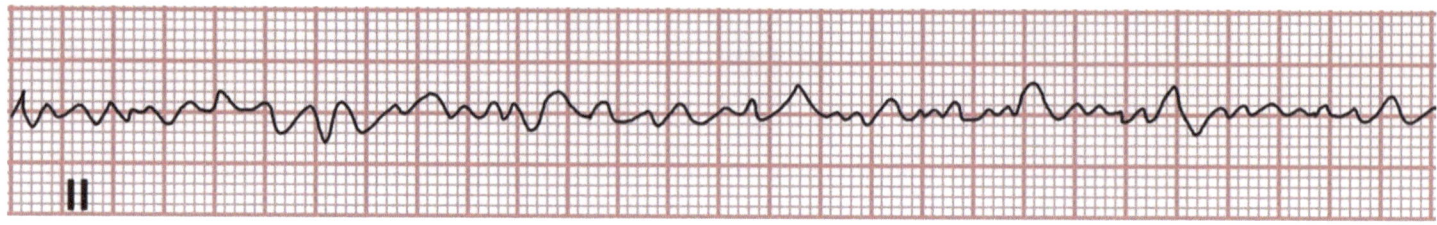

FIGURE 5 – 14: VENTRICULAR FIBRILLATION

Etiology:

This is caused by multiple automaticity foci in the ventricle, which stimulate the ventricles to contract at a faster rate and irregular rhythm. Here, the multiple automaticity foci fire chaotically, stimulating the ventricle to contract irregularly (unlike Ventricular tachycardia, which has a regular rhythm). Ventricular fibrillation is life-threatening because the ventricular contractions it produces are rapid but weak. These weak ventricular contractions are not strong enough to push an adequate amount of blood out of the ventricles. As a result, there is very low or no cardiac output, leading to the cessation of blood circulation. The lack of blood circulation causes pulselessness, low blood pressure, and loss of consciousness.

Causes: (HEAT DRUGS):
H Heart disorders like cardiomyopathy, aortic stenosis
E Electrolyte disorders: Hypokalemia, hypomagnesemia
A Acute myocardial infarction (especially within the first 24 hr.).
T Torsades de pointes.
Drugs that prolong QT interval: **ABCDE**
     Anti-**A**rrhythmia class **1**A, **3** (13 Friday the 13th)
     Anti-**B**iotic: Macrolide: Azithromycin, Clarithromycin, and Erythromycin
     Anti-Psy**C**hotic: Haloperidol
     Anti-**D**epressant: Tricyclic Antidepressant (TCA)
     Anti-**E**metic: Ondansetron

EKG findings:
Rate: Tachycardia
Rhythm: Irregular
P wave: None
PR interval: None
QRS: Varying width and height (Chaotic)

Clinical Features: PUB
P Pulseless
U Unconscious
B BP Low (Hypotensive)

Treatment:
Follow the ACLS flow chart

ACLS Flow chart:

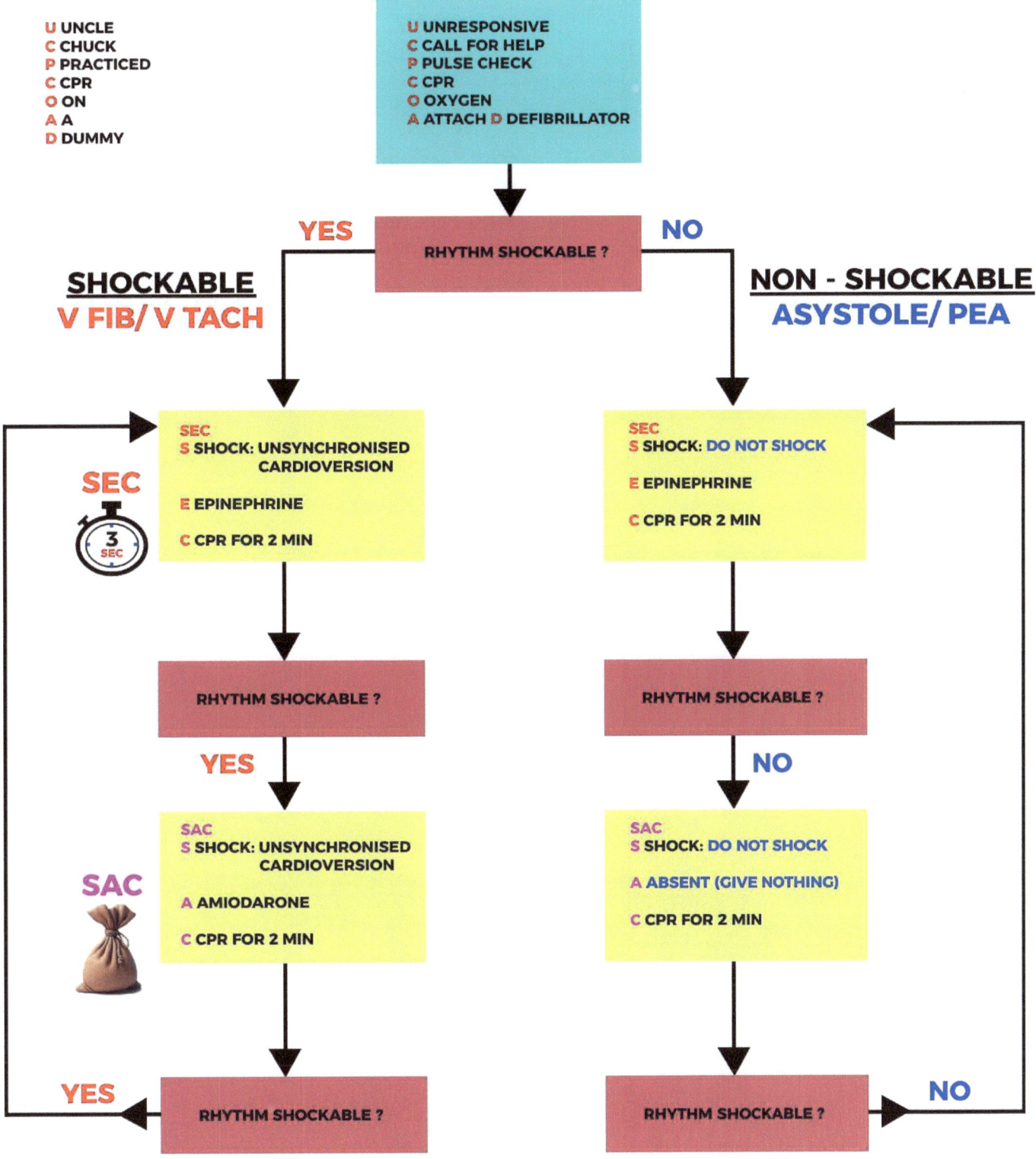

FIGURE 5 – 15: ACLS TREATMENT FLOWCHART FOR VENTRICULAR FIBRILLATION

FIGURE 5 – 16: VENTRICULAR FIBRILLATION

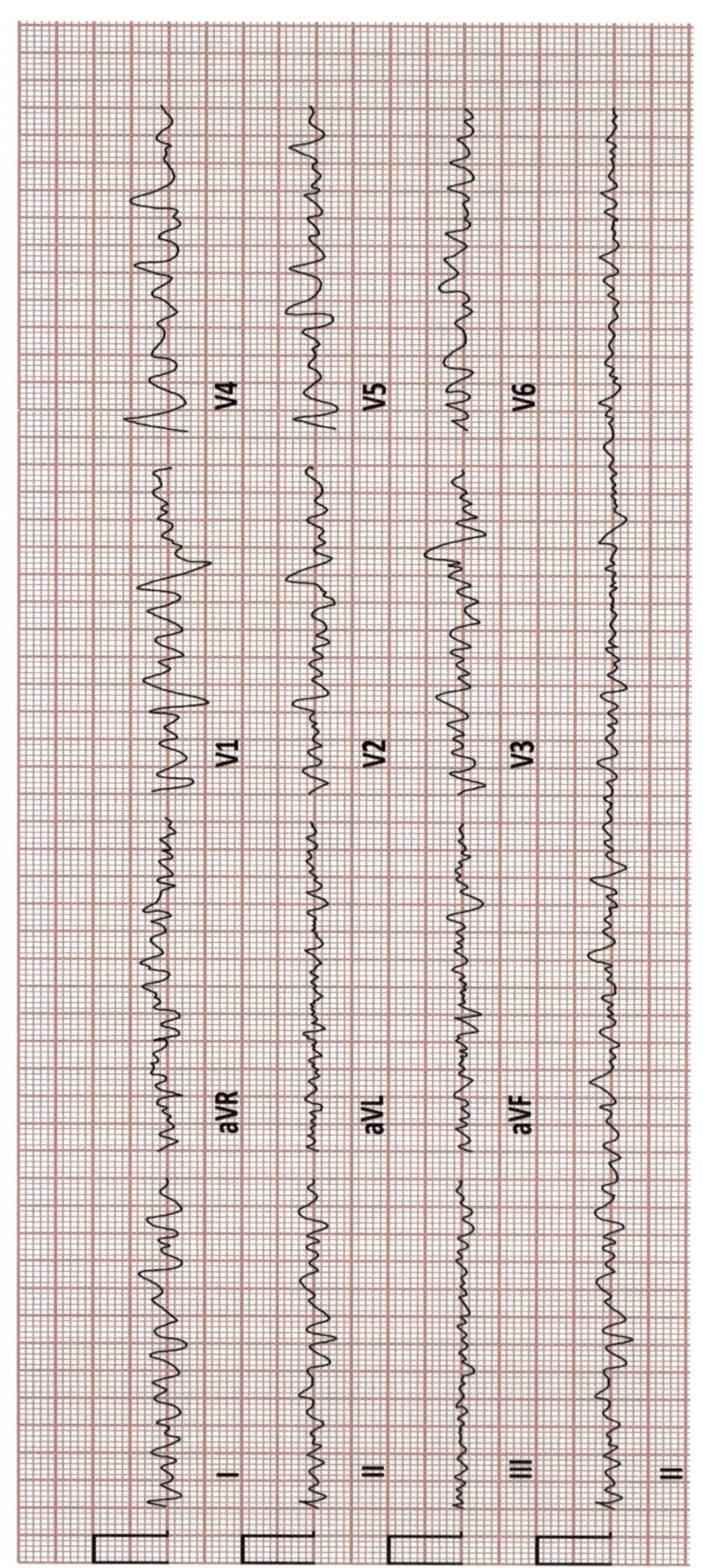

EKG findings:
Rate: Tachycardia
Rhythm: Irregular
P wave: None
PR interval: None
QRS: Varying width and height (Chaotic)

Question 9:

An 87-year-old female patient suddenly loses consciousness in front of you while walking to the bathroom. You called for help and started CPR. Her telemetry monitor displays the following image below. How would you treat this patient?

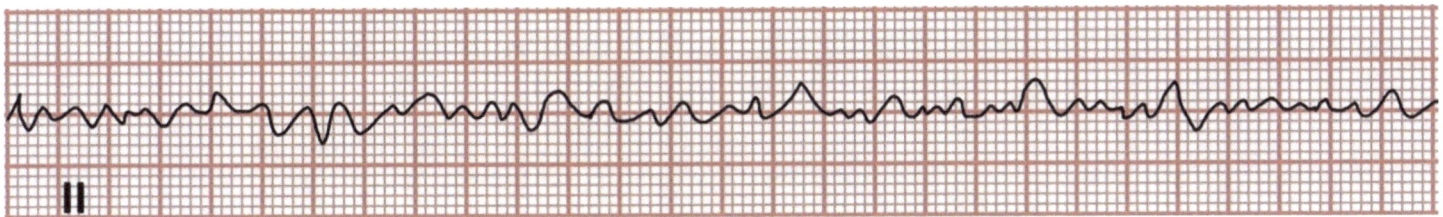

A. Unsynchronized cardioversion
B. Synchronized Cardioversion

Question 9: The answer is B. Unsynchronized cardioversion. Remember the earlier mnemonic: You only use synchronized cardioversion with the man standing in the "sink" with unstable clinical features. This patient does not have any unstable clinical features. The Telemetry EKG shows ventricular fibrillation. Using the ACLS flow chart, ventricular fibrillation is a shockable rhythm, and the treatment is unsynchronized cardioversion.

MULTIFOCAL ATRIAL TACHYCARDIA (MFAT)

Single EKG strip

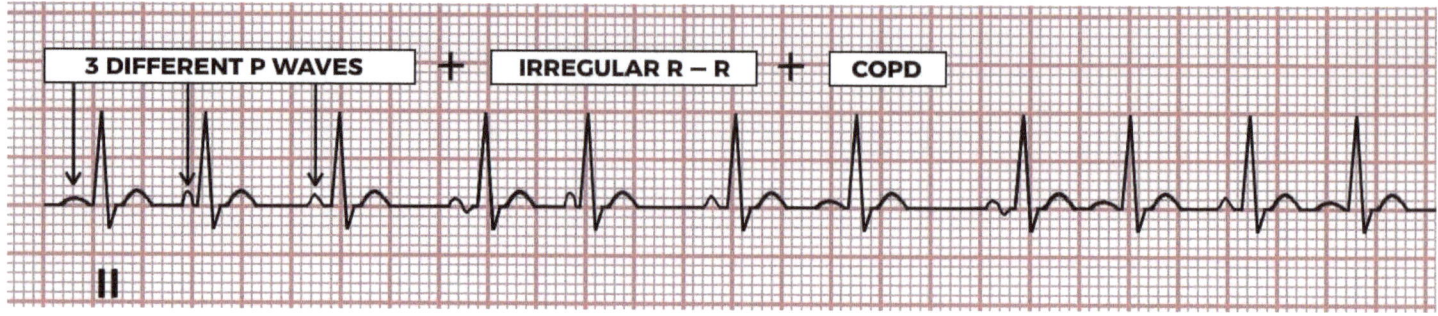

FIGURE 5 – 17: MULTIFOCAL ATRIAL TACHYCARDIA

Etiology:
There are multiple automaticity foci located in the atrium, and each of them stimulates the atrium to contract. Since there are multiple automaticity foci stimulating the atrium, each focus produces its own distinct P wave, resulting in a rhythm in which at least 3 consecutive P waves are different from each other. This arrhythmia is classically seen in elderly patients with COPD.

Causes:
COPD

EKG findings:
Rate: Tachycardia
Rhythm: Irregular
P wave: Each new p wave is different from the last one
PR interval: PR interval is variable (not constant)
QRS: Normal

(Note: The arrhythmia wandering pacemaker has the same etiology and clinical features as multifocal atrial tachycardia, the only difference is that the heart rate in wandering pacemaker is less than 100 BPM, and in multifocal atrial tachycardia, the heart rate is greater than 100 BPM)

Clinical Features:
COPD
Elderly
+
P Pulse: Tachycardia + irregular
P Palpitation

Lab:
Best initial test: EKG

Treatment:
Definitive treatment: Treat COPD
Avoid Beta blocker

FIGURE 5 – 18: MULTIFOCAL ATRIAL TACHYCARDIA

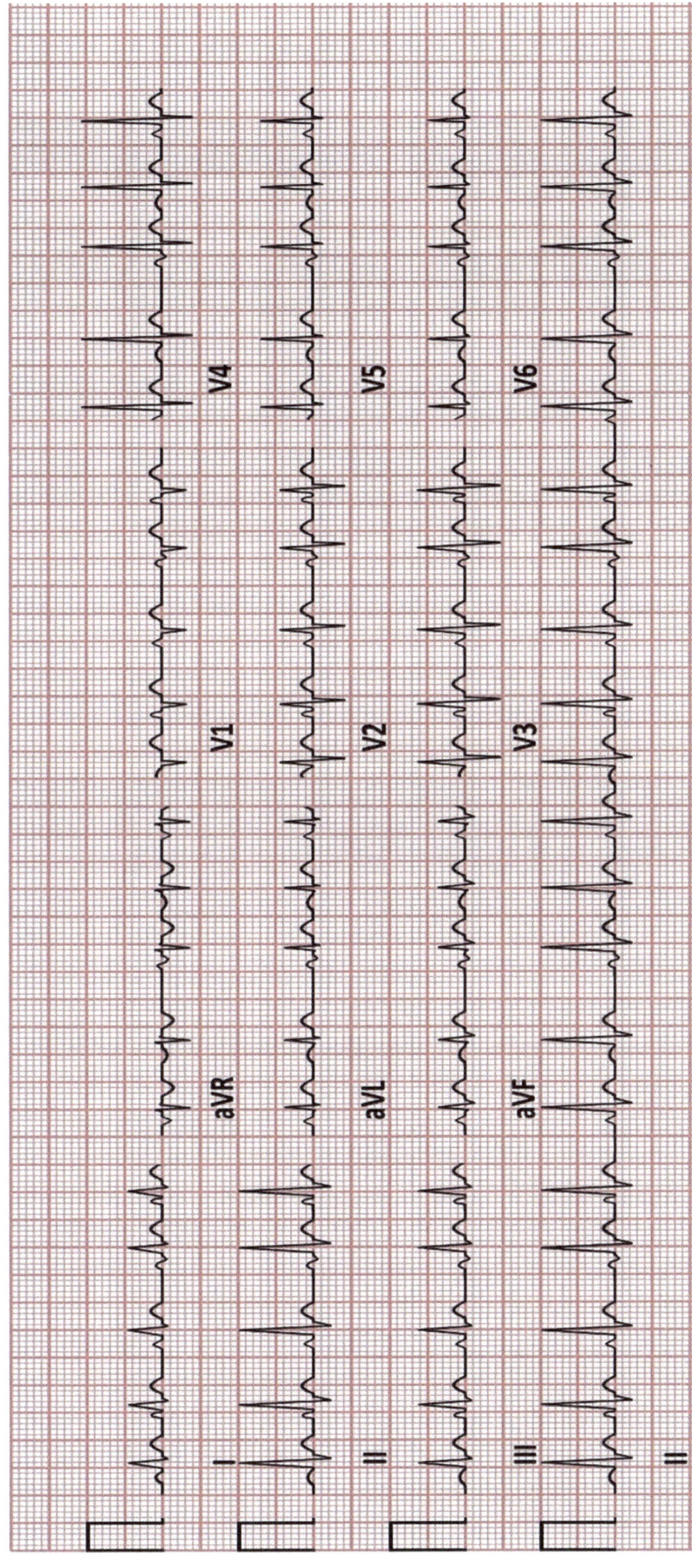

EKG findings:
Rate: Tachycardia
Rhythm: Irregular
P wave: Each new p wave is different
PR interval: PR interval is variable (not constant)
QRS: Normal

ATRIAL FIBRILLATION

Single EKG strip

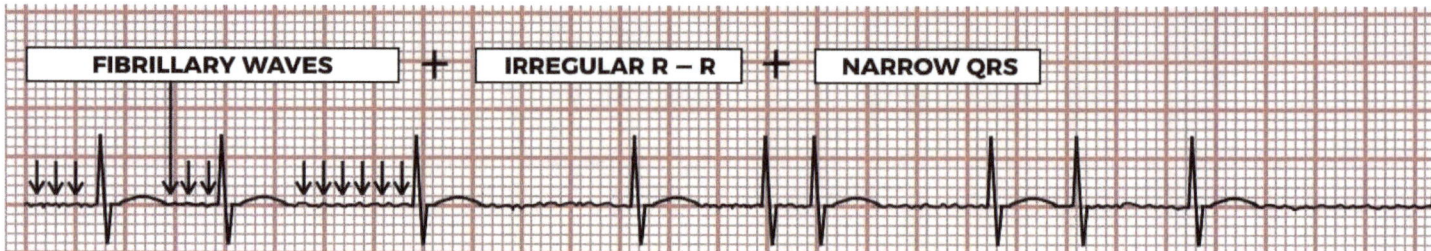

FIGURE 5 – 19: ATRIAL FIBRILLATION

Etiology:
This is caused by multiple automaticity foci in the atria, which stimulate the atria to contract at a faster rate and irregular rhythm. Here, the automaticity foci fire chaotically, stimulating the atria to contract irregularly (unlike atrial flutter, which has a regular rhythm). These irregular contractions produce fibrillary waves which have different heights and widths and are irregularly spaced. The fibrillary waves may be so tiny that they appear as straight lines on the EKG. Atrial fibrillation can cause heart failure by decreasing ventricular filling. This occurs due to a decrease in filling time in the atrium, which will cause a reduction in cardiac Output.

Causes: HAM
H Hyperthyroidism
A Anemia
M Mitral stenosis

EKG findings:
Rate: Tachycardia
Rhythm: Irregular
P wave: NO P WAVES, only fibrillary waves (tiny uneven spiky waves)
PR interval: None
QRS: Narrow QRS
+
Fibrillary waves: These are tiny, uneven, spiky waves. The waves have different heights and widths and are irregularly spaced.
(Note: flutter waves seen in atrial flutter are identical with the same height and width)

Once a patient has Atrial fibrillation with a heart rate > 100 BPM, then the diagnosis changes from atrial fibrillation to **atrial fibrillation with Rapid Ventricular Response (RVR).**

Clinical Features:
Asymptomatic: Most patients are asymptomatic
OR
Symptomatic
Fatigue
Lightheadedness
P Palpitation
P Pulse: Tachycardia and Irregularly Irregular
OR
Unilateral muscle weakness + pulse irregularly irregular (A Fib patients in vignettes sometimes present with a stroke)

Lab:
Best initial test: EKG
Transthoracic Echocardiography
CMP, CBC, Chest X-ray, Thyroid function test

Treatment:
If moderate or severe mitral valve disease is present:
A Anticoagulant: **Warfarin MUST be used if moderate or severe mitral valve disease is present**
R Rate control: Both Calcium Channel Blockers: Diltiazem, or Beta Blocker: Metoprolol are **1st line**
R Rhythm control: Amiodarone

No mitral valve disease:
A Anticoagulant: **Aspirin, Novel anticoagulant (NAC), or Warfarin** (depending on the CHADS Score)
  d. CHADS Score of 0 = No Anticoagulant required

  e. CHADS Score of 1 = Give Aspirin, Warfarin or Novel anticoagulant: Dabigatran, Rivaroxaban, Apixaban

  f. CHADS Score of ≥ 2 = Give Warfarin or Novel anticoagulant: Dabigatran, Rivaroxaban, Apixaban (Never give Aspirin when the CHAD Score is equal to or greater than 2)

R Rate control: Both Calcium Channel Blockers: Diltiazem, or Beta Blocker: Metoprolol are **1st line**
R Rhythm control: Amiodarone

CHADS Score:
The whole point of calculating the CHADS score is that the number you obtain at the end of the calculation will be used to select an anticoagulant to be given to the patient with Atrial Fibrillation.

CHADS VAS

CRITERIA	POINTS
C CHF	1
H HTN	1
A Age > 75 *	1
A Age > 75 *	1
D DM	1
S Stroke/ TIA	1
S Stroke/ TIA	1
V Vascular disease: CAD	1
A Age 65 – 75 *	1
S Sex: Female	1
TOTAL	9

CHF = Congestive Heart failure; **HTN** = Hypertension;
DM = Diabetes Mellitus; **TIA** = Transient Ischemic Attack; **CAD** = Coronary Artery Disease.
* = If the patient's age is between 65 – 75 years, they score 1 point, but if the patients age is > 75 years they score 2 points.

FIGURE 5 – 20: FIGURE 2 – 1: ATRIAL FIBRILLATION

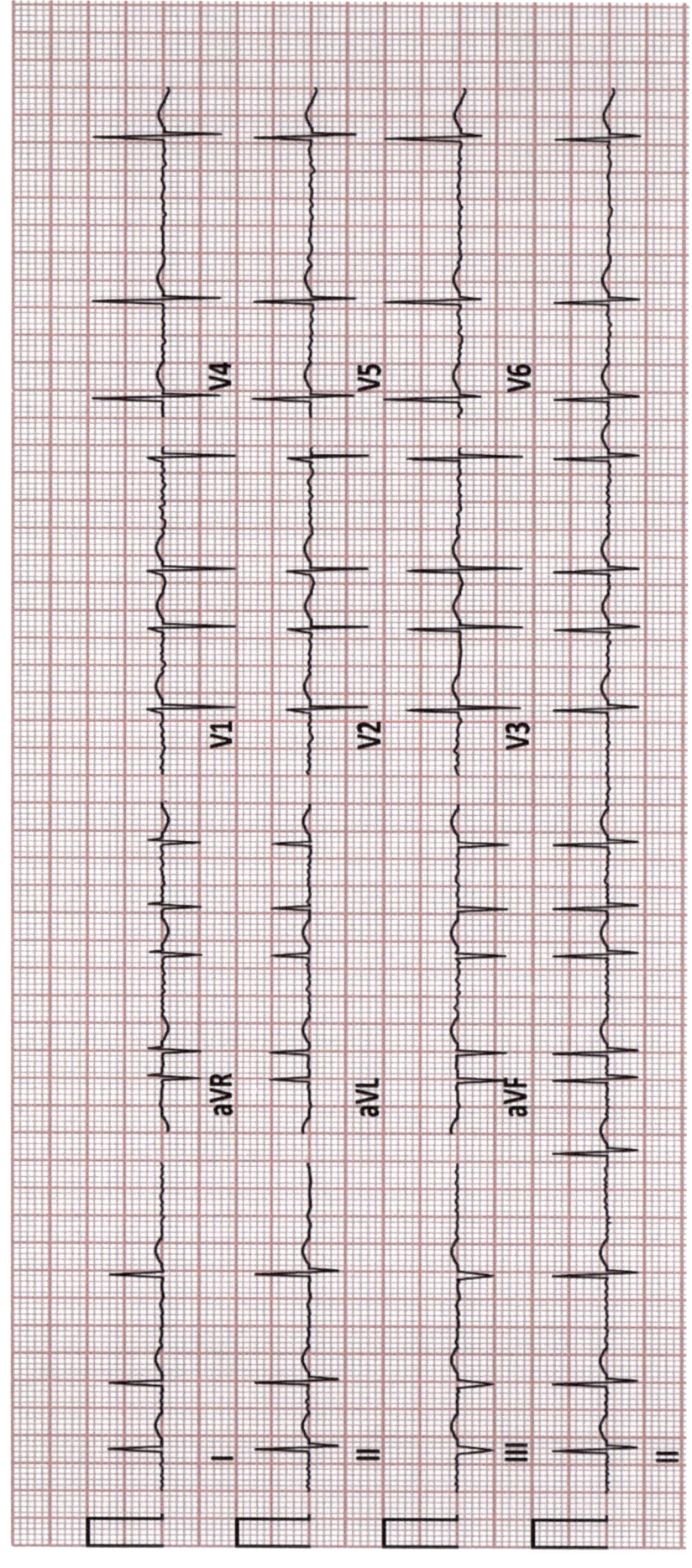

EKG findings:
Rate: Tachycardia
Rhythm: Irregular
P wave: NO P WAVES, only fibrillary waves (tiny uneven spiky waves)
PR interval: None
QRS: Narrow QRS
+
Fibrillary waves: These are tiny, uneven, spiky waves. The waves have different heights and widths and are irregularly spaced.

Question 10:
A 76-year-old female comes to the ER complaining of palpitations. She has had hypertension for 10 years. On examination, her pulse is irregularly irregular. An EKG shows atrial fibrillation with a pulse rate of 135 BPM; what is the best initial treatment?
   A. Amiodarone
   B. Metoprolol

Question 10: The answer is B, Metoprolol. This patient's heart rate is elevated at 135 BPM. So for this patient with atrial fibrillation, the rate control is managed first with a beta blocker such as Metoprolol, before managing the rhythm control with Amiodarone.

Bradycardia + Regular Arrhythmias:

SINUS BRADYCARDIA

Single EKG strip

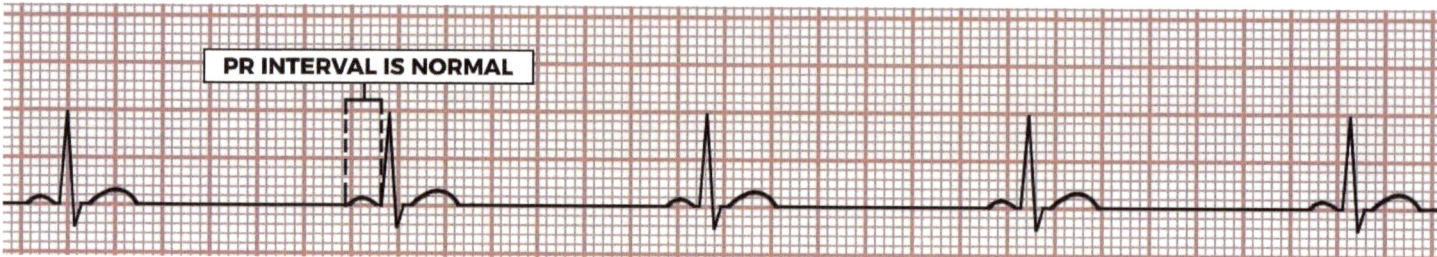

FIGURE 5 – 21: SINUS BRADYCARDIA

Etiology:
This is caused by the SA node firing at less than 60 BPM.

Causes: **R**ed **B**lood **C**ell + **Ha**
R Right coronary artery myocardial infarction (Right coronary artery supplies the SA node)
B Beta blockers
C Calcium channel blockers
+
H Hypothyroidism
A Athletic history

EKG findings:
Rate: Bradycardia
Rhythm: Regular
P wave: Normal. The P wave is present before every QRS.
PR interval: Normal
QRS: Normal
(Note: the difference between first-degree heart block and sinus bradycardia is that, in sinus bradycardia, the PR interval is normal, but in first-degree heart block, the PR interval is prolonged)

Clinical Features:
Asymptomatic
OR
Symptomatic
PHD
P Pulse: Bradycardia and regular
P Palpitation
H Hypotension
D Dizziness/ Lightheadedness

Lab:
Best initial test: EKG

Treatment:
   A. **Asymptomatic:**
      Reassurance

   B. **Symptomatic:**
      Best initial treatment: Atropine

FIGURE 5 – 22: SINUS BRADYCARDIA

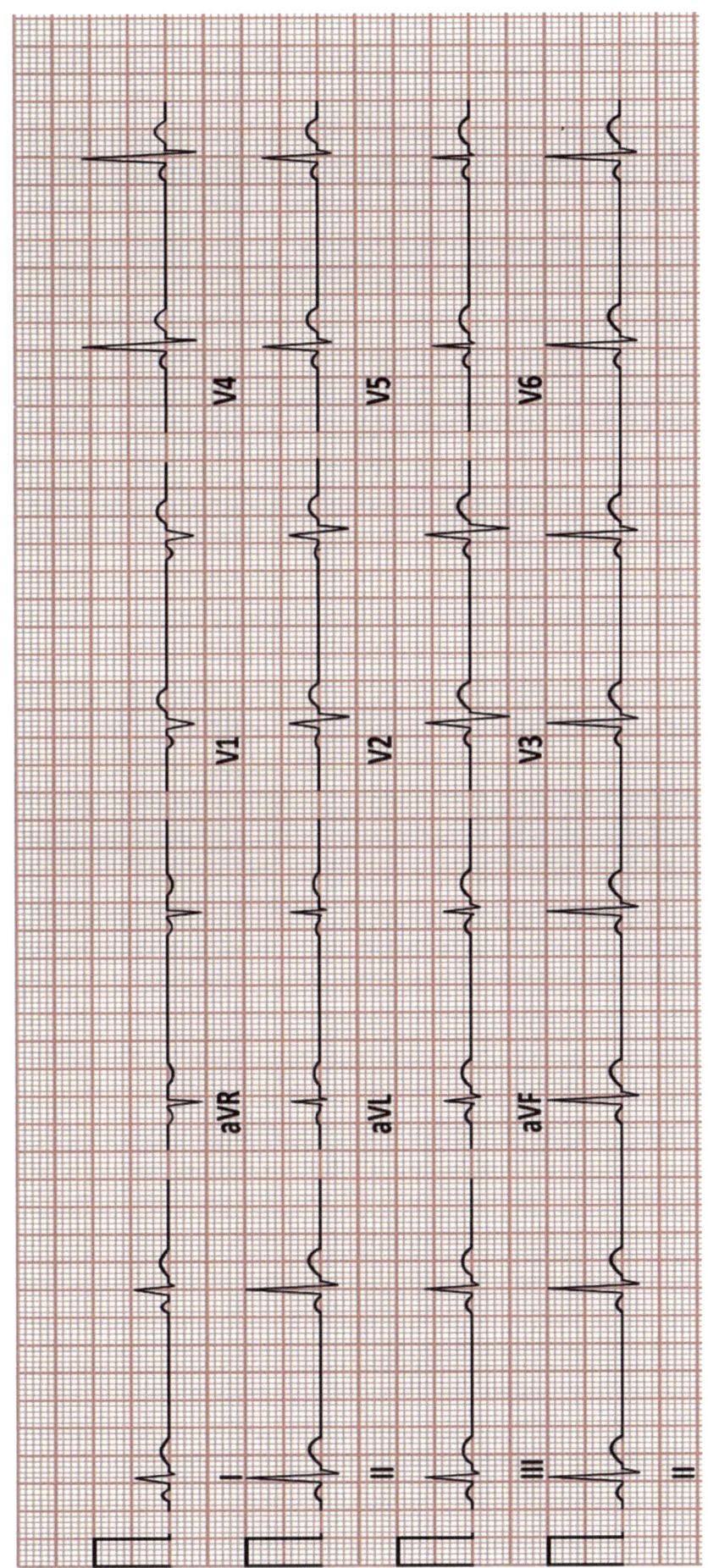

EKG Findings:
Rate: Bradycardia
Rhythm: Regular
P wave: Normal. The P wave is present before every QRS.
PR interval: Normal
QRS: Normal

FIRST-DEGREE HEART BLOCK

Single EKG strip

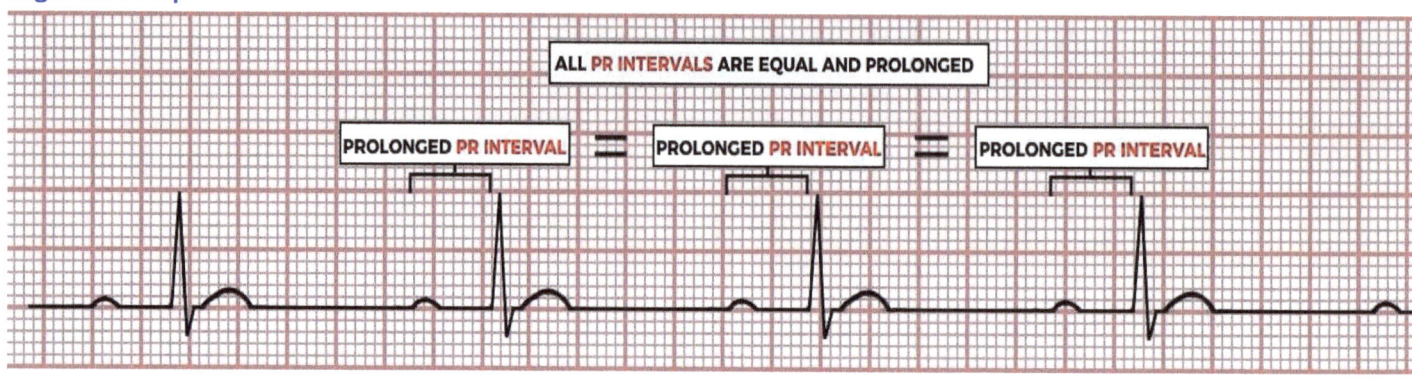

FIGURE 5 – 23: FIRST-DEGREE HEART BLOCK

Etiology:
This is caused by an abnormality of the AV node. This is due to an abnormal electrical conduction delay of impulses passing through the AV node, resulting in a prolonged PR interval.

Causes: RBC
R Right coronary artery myocardial infarction (Right coronary artery supplies the AV node)
B Beta blockers
C Calcium channel blockers

EKG findings:
Rate: Bradycardia
Rhythm: Regular P – P intervals and Regular R – R intervals
P wave: Normal. P waves are present before every QRS
PR interval: Prolonged (greater than 200 ms or 0.2 sec)
QRS: Normal
NO DROPPED QRS
(Note: To differentiate first and third-degree heart blocks from both second-degree heart blocks, there is no dropped QRS in the first and third-degree heart blocks, but in both second-degree heart blocks, the QRS is dropped)

Clinical Features:
Asymptomatic
OR
Symptomatic: PHD
P Pulse: Bradycardia and regular
P Palpitation
H Hypotension
D Dizziness/ Lightheadedness

Lab:
Best initial test: EKG

Treatment:
   A. **Asymptomatic**
      Observe and reassure

   B. **Symptomatic:**
      Best initial treatment: Atropine

FIGURE 5 – 24: FIRSR DEGREE HEART BLOCK

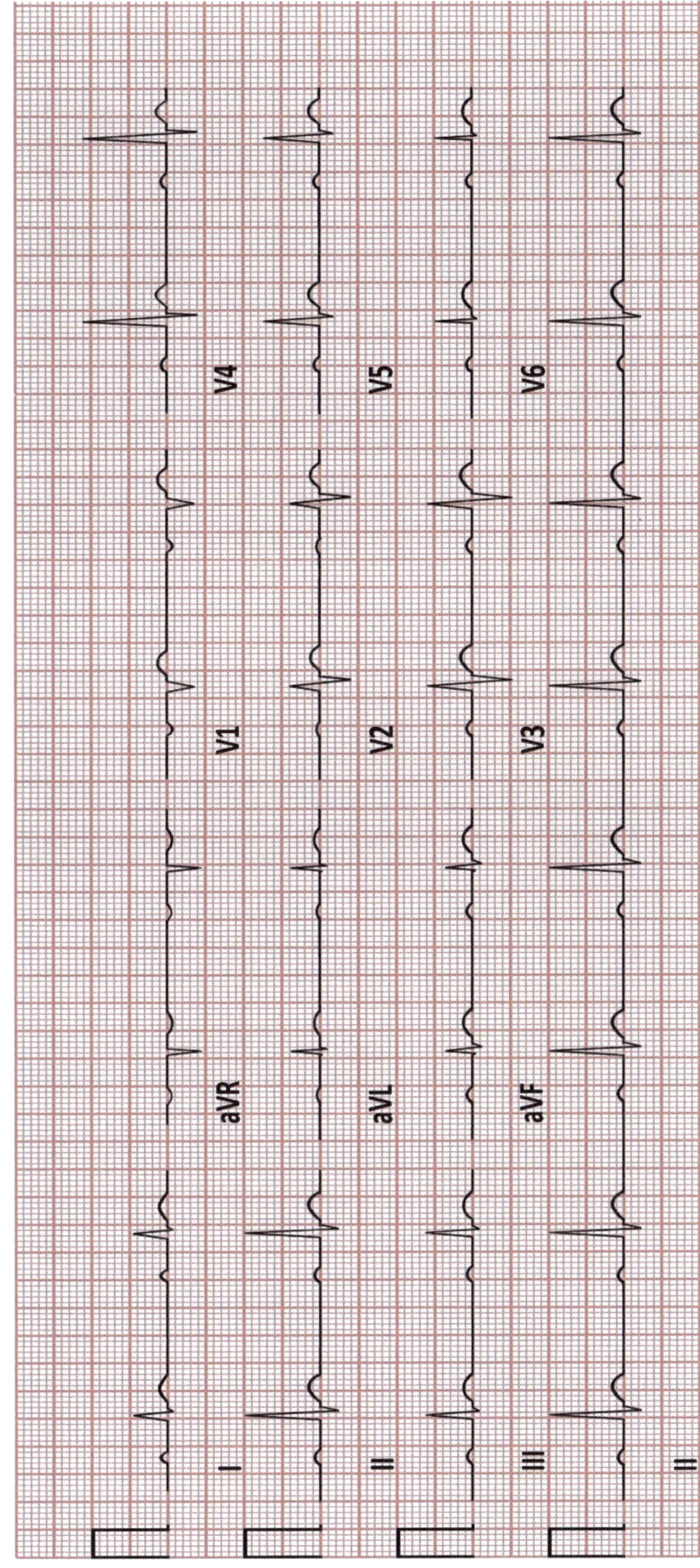

EKG findings:
Rate: Bradycardia
Rhythm: Regular P – P intervals and Regular R –R intervals
P wave: Normal. P waves are present before every QRS
PR interval: Prolonged (greater than 200 ms or 0.2 sec)
QRS: Normal
NO DROPPED QRS

THIRD-DEGREE HEART BLOCK

Single EKG strip

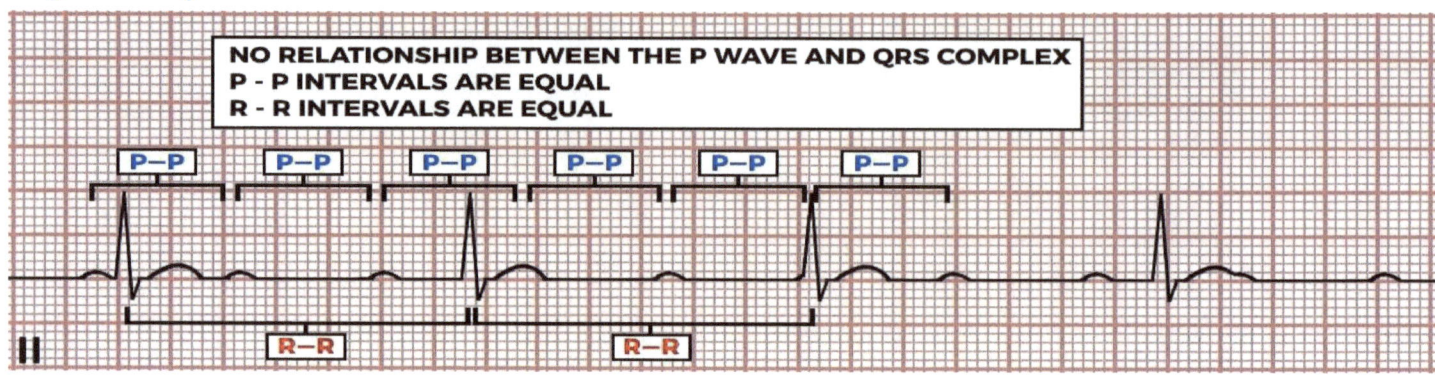

FIGURE 5 – 25: THIRD-DEGREE HEART BLOCK

Etiology:
This is caused by an abnormality of the AV node. The Impulses generated from the SA node are **completely** blocked from passing through the AV node to reach the ventricles. Due to this blockage, an accessory pacemaker develops in the ventricles and stimulates the ventricles to contract independently of the SA node's stimulation. So, the atrium beats independently from the ventricle. The atrium beats faster than the ventricle, and you will see more P waves than QRS waves on the EKG.

Causes: RBC + LA
R Right coronary artery myocardial infarction (Right coronary artery supplies the AV node)
B Beta blockers
C Calcium channel blockers
+
L Lyme disease
A Ankylosis spondylitis

EKG findings:
Rate: Bradycardia
Rhythm: Regular P – P intervals and regular R – R interval
P wave: P wave is not related to QRS. They are both produced independently of each other.
PR interval: It varies and is prolonged (greater than 200 ms)
QRS: Normal + **NO DROPPED QRS**
(Note: To differentiate first and third-degree heart blocks from both second-degree heart blocks, there is no dropped QRS in the first and third-degree heart blocks, but in both second-degree heart blocks, the QRS is dropped)

Clinical Features:
Asymptomatic
OR
Symptomatic PHD
P Pulse: Bradycardia and regular
P Palpitation
H Hypotension
D Dizziness/ Lightheadedness

Lab:
Best initial test: EKG

Treatment:
A. **Symptomatic or asymptomatic:**
   A pacemaker is the **only** treatment, even if the patient is asymptomatic
   Never give Atropine. Atropine **is always wrong.**

FIGURE 5 – 26: THIRD-DEGREE HEART BLOCK

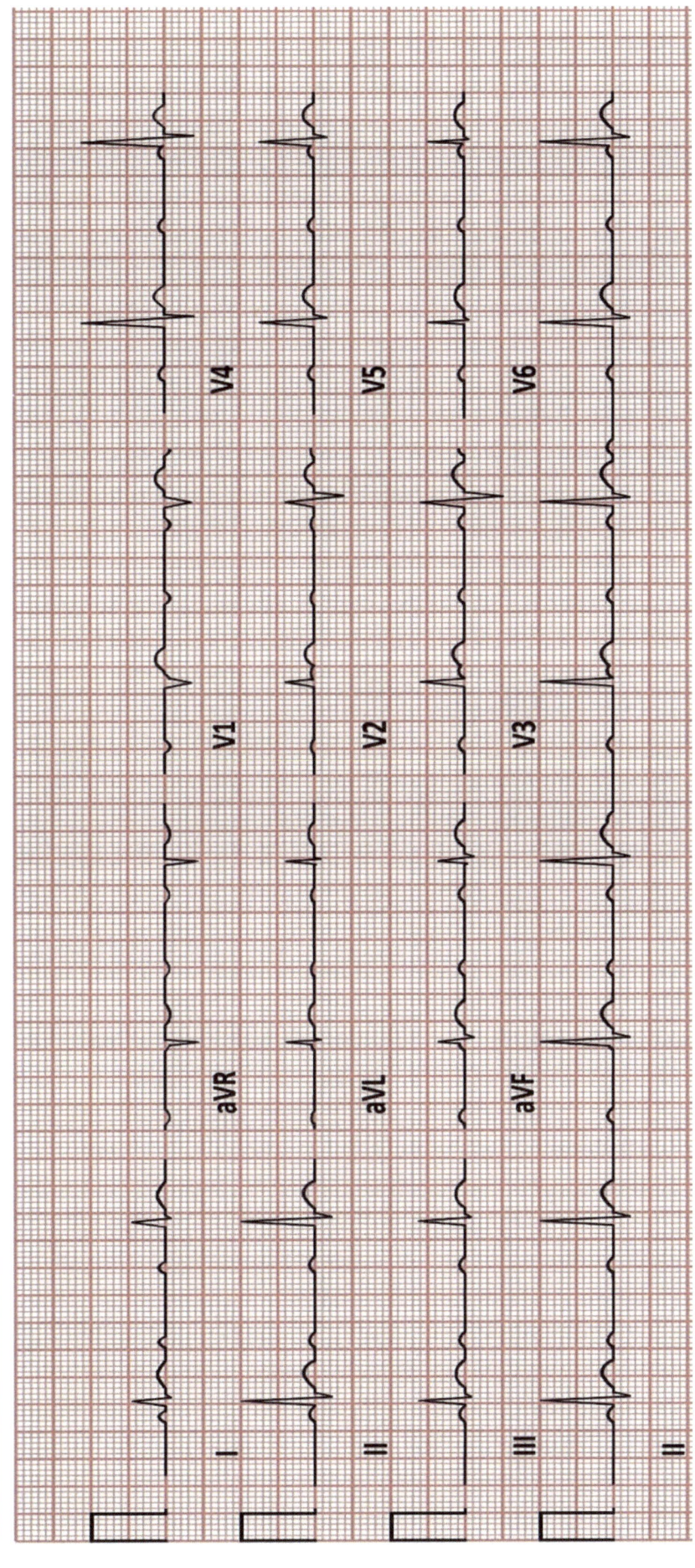

EKG findings:
Rate: Bradycardia
Rhythm: Regular P – P intervals and regular R –R interval
P wave: P wave is not related to QRS. They are both produced independently of each other.
PR interval: It varies and is prolonged (greater than 200 ms)
QRS: Normal
NO DROPPED QRS

Bradycardia + Irregular Arrhythmias:

SECOND-DEGREE HEART BLOCK TYPE 1 (WENCKEBACH OR MOBITZ TYPE 1)

Single EKG strip

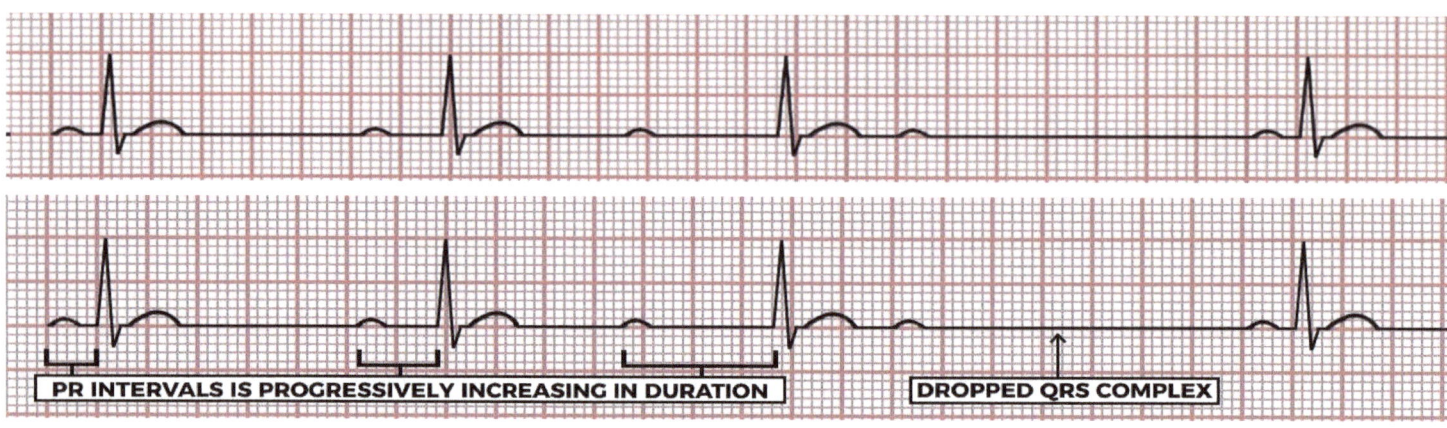

FIGURE 5 – 27: SECOND-DEGREE HEART BLOCK TYPE 1

Etiology:
This is caused by an abnormality of the AV node. The AV node is incompletely blocked. The impulses generated by the SA node are abnormally slowed down by the AV node before passing to the ventricles. It is harder for impulses to pass through the AV node to reach the ventricles.

Causes: RBC
R Right coronary artery myocardial infarction (Right coronary artery supplies the AV node)
B Beta blockers
C Calcium channel blockers

EKG findings:
Rate: Bradycardia
Rhythm: Irregular
P wave: Upright
PR interval: Prolonged (greater than 200ms). The PR interval keeps **PROLONGING till the QRS drops.**
QRS: Normal
(Note: the difference between second-degree heart block type 1 and type 2 is that in type 1, the PR interval keeps prolonging till the QRS is dropped, but in type 2, the PR interval is constant, and the QRS drops randomly)

Clinical Features:
Asymptomatic
OR
Symptomatic PHD
P Pulse: Bradycardia and regular
P Palpitation
H Hypotension
D Dizziness/ Lightheadedness

Lab:
Best initial test: EKG

Treatment:
A. **Asymptomatic**
   Observe and reassure
B. **Symptomatic:**
   Best initial treatment: Atropine
   Definitive treatment: Pacemaker

FIGURE 5 – 28: SECOND-DEGREE HEART BLOCK TYPE 1

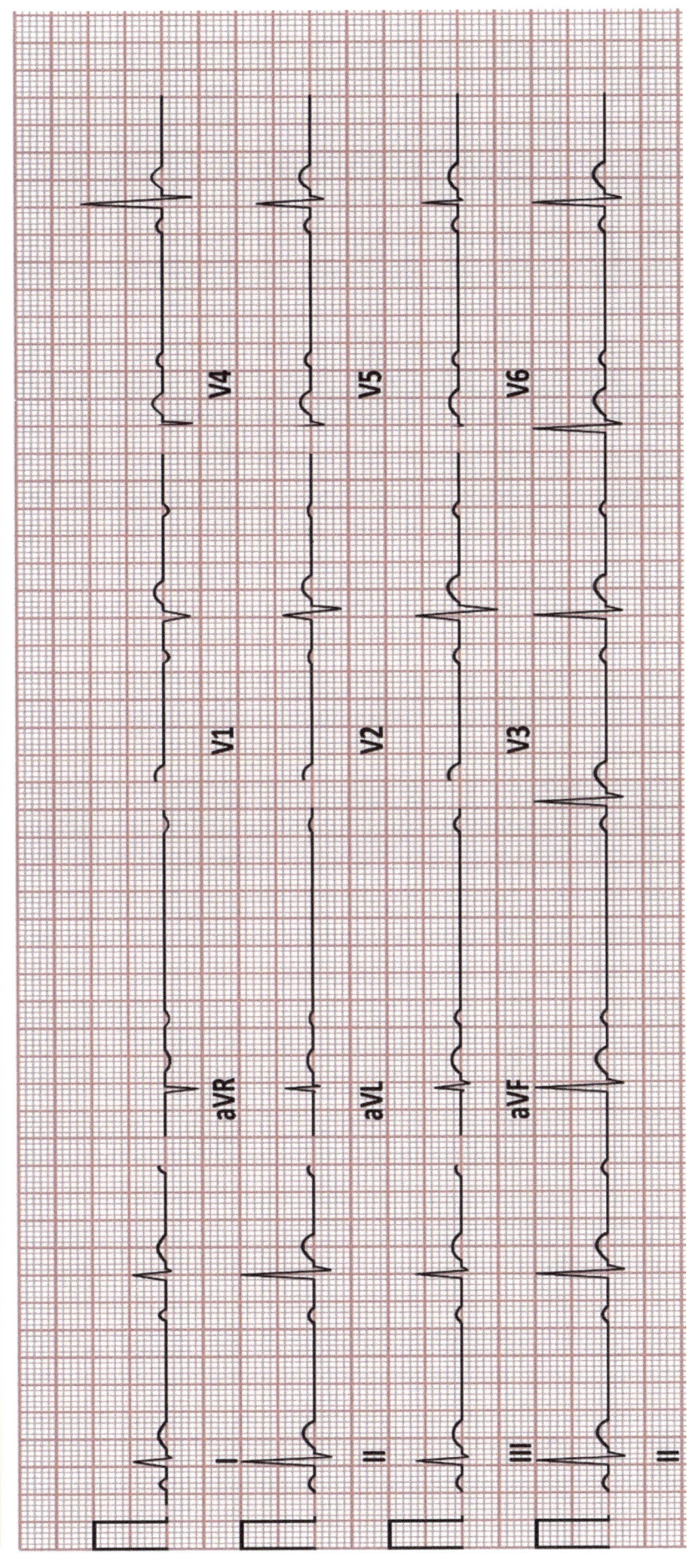

EKG findings:
Rate: Bradycardia
Rhythm: Irregular
P wave: Upright
PR interval: Prolonged (greater than 200ms). The PR interval keeps **PROLONGING till the QRS drops.**
QRS: Normal

SECOND-DEGREE HEART BLOCK TYPE 2 (MORBITZ OR MORBITZ TYPE 2)

Single EKG strip

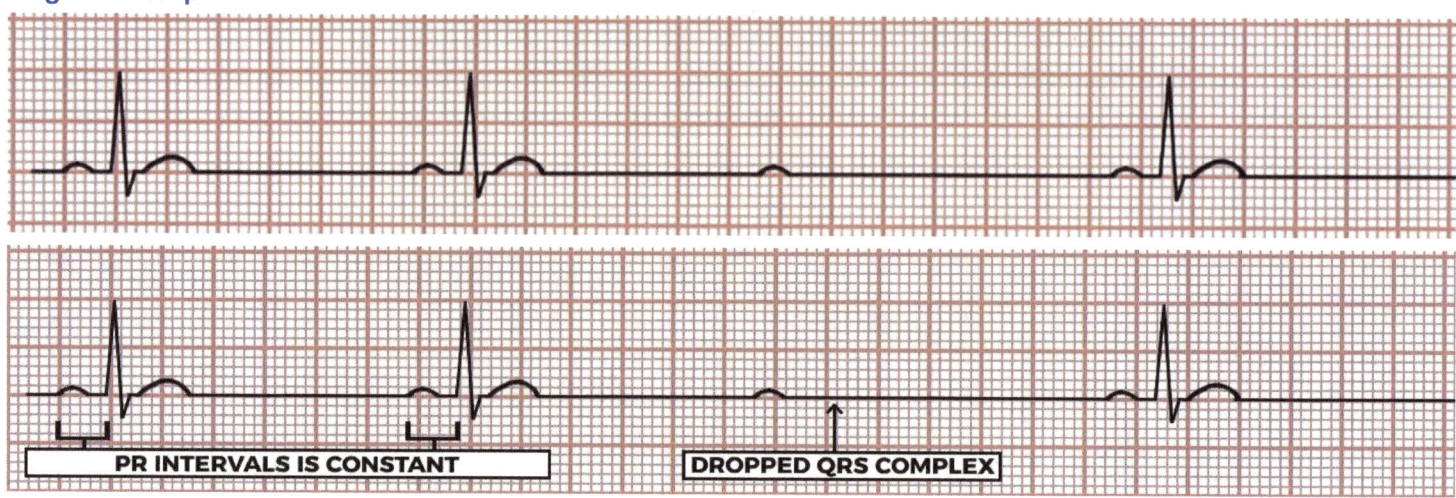

FIGURE 5 – 29: SECOND-DEGREE HEART BLOCK TYPE 2

Etiology:
This is caused by an abnormality of the AV node. The AV node is incompletely blocked. The impulses generated by the SA node are abnormally slowed down by the AV node before passing to the ventricles. It is harder for impulses to pass through the AV node to reach the ventricles.

Causes: RBC
R Right coronary artery myocardial infarction (Right coronary artery supplies the AV node)
B Beta blockers
C Calcium channel blockers

EKG findings:
Rate: Bradycardia
Rhythm: Regular P – P intervals and Irregular R –R intervals
P wave: Normal
PR interval: Prolonged (greater than 200 ms). The PR interval is constant, and the **QRS drops randomly**.
QRS: Normal
(Note: the difference between second-degree heart block type 1 and type 2 is that in type 1, the PR interval keeps prolonging till the QRS is dropped, but in type 2, the PR interval is constant, and the QRS drops randomly)

Clinical Features:
Asymptomatic
OR
Symptomatic PHD
P Pulse: Bradycardia and regular
P Palpitation
H Hypotension
D Dizziness/ Lightheadedness

Lab:
Best initial test: EKG

Treatment:
A. **Symptomatic or asymptomatic:**
   A pacemaker is the **only** treatment, even if the patient is asymptomatic
   Never give Atropine. Atropine **is always wrong.**

FIGURE 5 – 30: SECOND-DEGREE HEART BLOCK TYPE 2

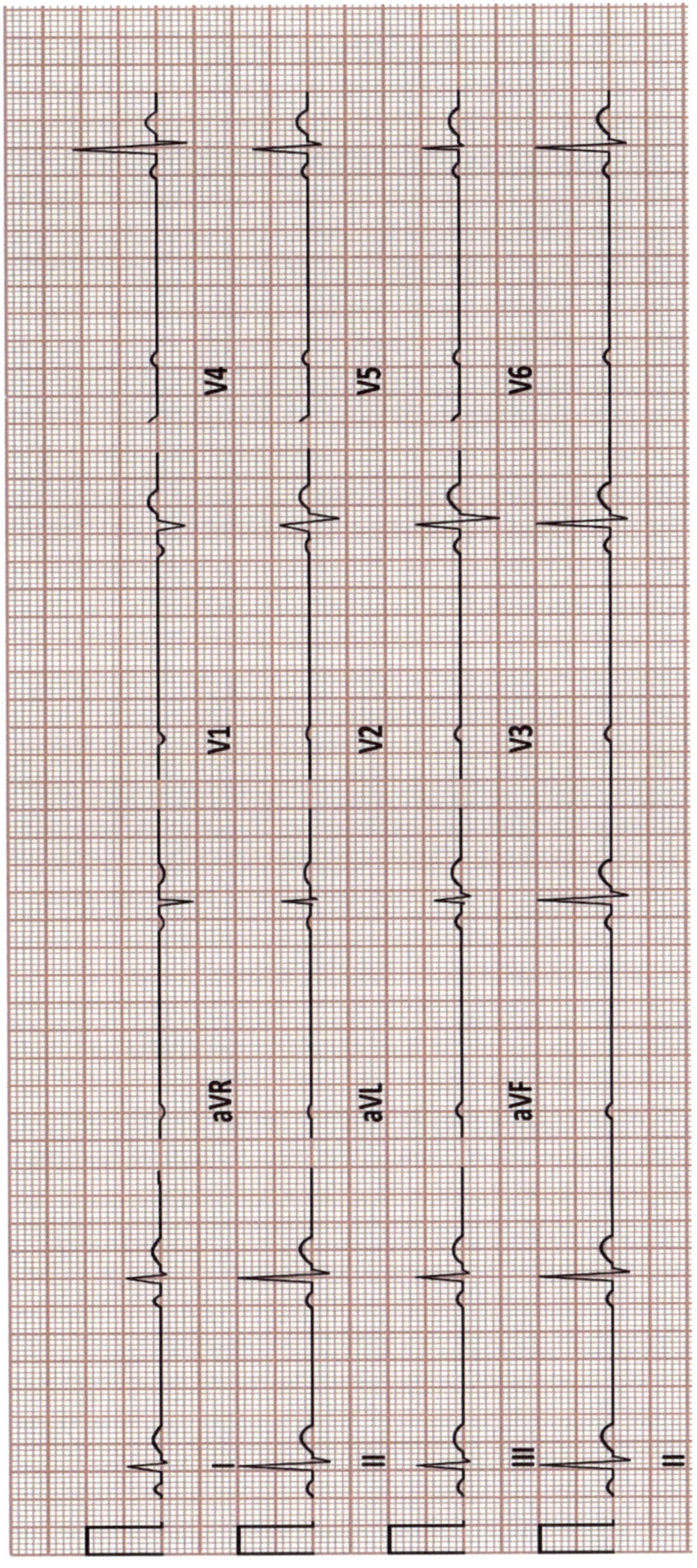

EKG findings:
Rate: Bradycardia
Rhythm: Regular P – P intervals and Irregular R –R intervals
P wave: Normal
PR interval: Prolonged (greater than 200 ms). The PR interval is constant, and the **QRS drops randomly.**
QRS: Normal

Normal rate + Irregular Arrhythmias:

WANDERING PACEMAKER:

Single EKG strip

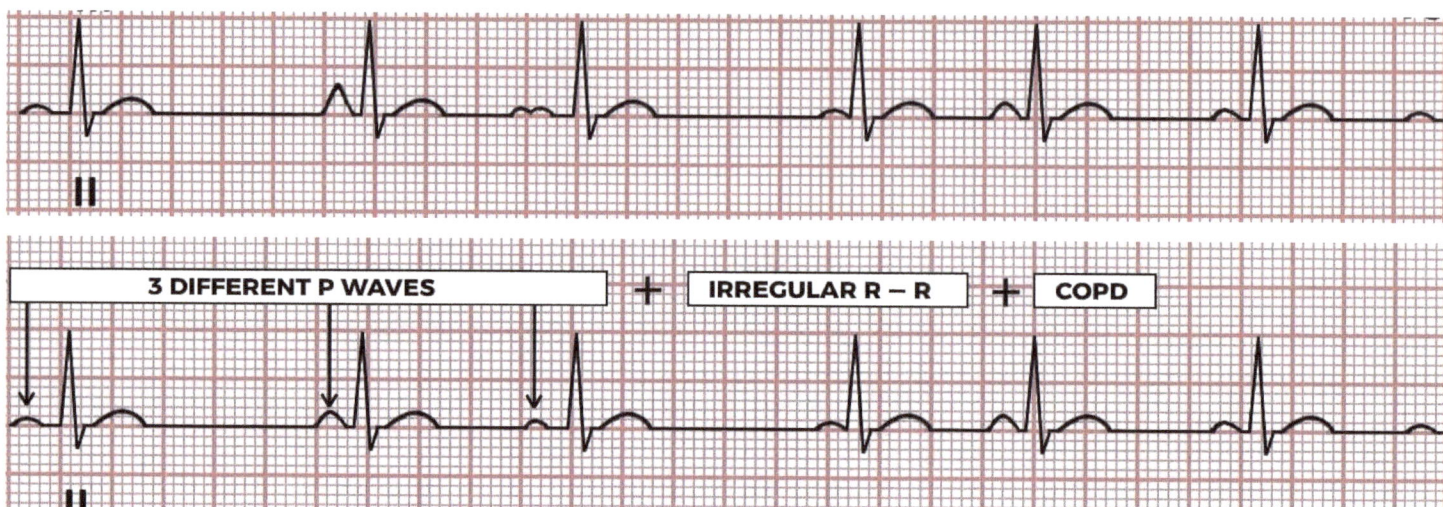

FIGURE 5 – 31: WANDERING PACEMAKER

Etiology:
There are multiple automaticity foci located in the atrium, and each of them stimulates the atrium to contract. Since there are multiple automaticity foci stimulating the atrium, each focus produces its own distinct P wave, resulting in a rhythm in which at least 3 consecutive P waves are different from each other. This arrhythmia is classically seen in elderly patients with COPD.

Causes:
COPD

EKG findings:
Rate: Normal
Rhythm: Irregular
P wave: Each new p wave is different from the last
PR interval: PR interval is variable (not constant)
QRS: Normal
(Note: The arrhythmia wandering pacemaker has the same etiology and clinical features as multifocal atrial tachycardia, the only difference is that the heart rate in wandering pacemaker is less than 100 BPM, and in multifocal atrial tachycardia, the heart rate is greater than 100 BPM)

Clinical Features:
COPD
Elderly
+
P Pulse: Normal rate + irregular
P Palpitation

Lab:
Best initial test: EKG

Treatment:
Definitive treatment: Treat COPD
Avoid Beta blocker

FIGURE 5 – 32: WANDERING PACEMAKER

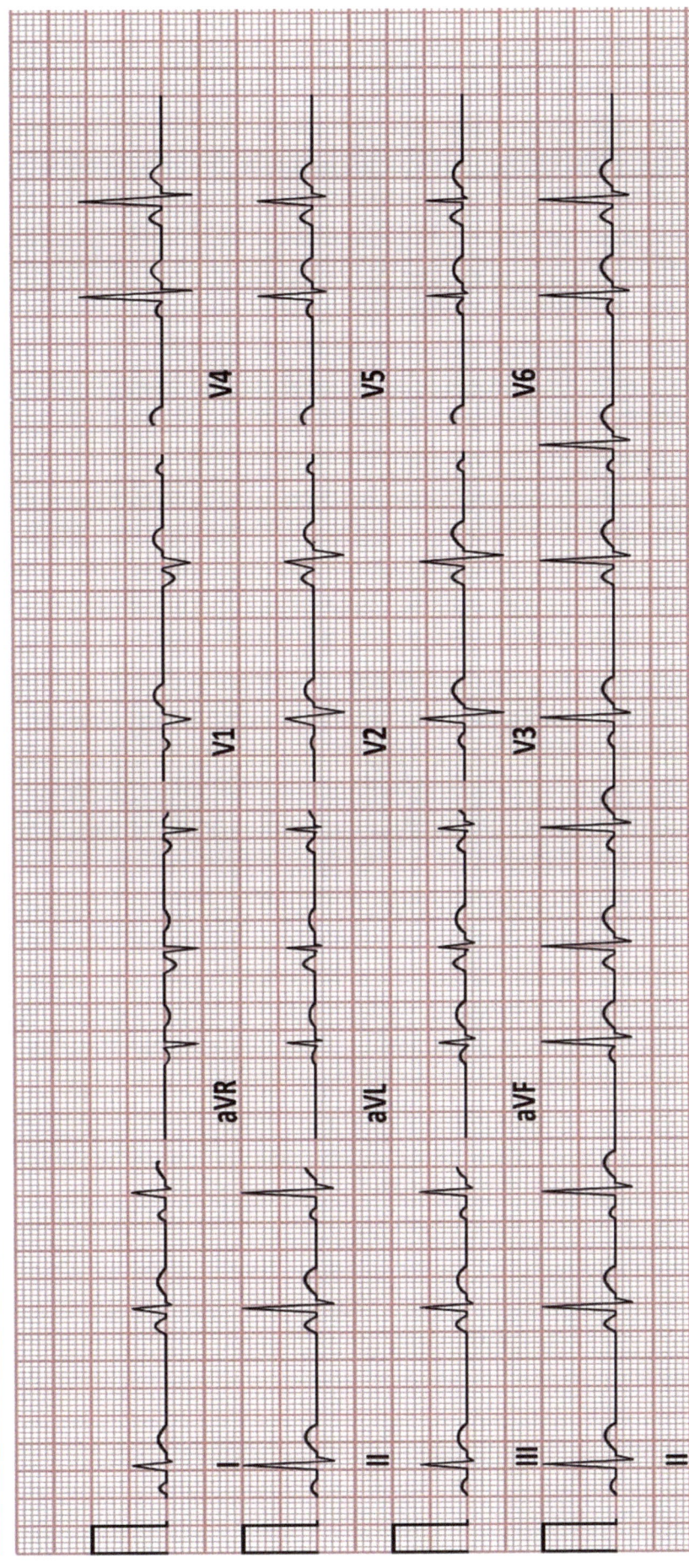

EKG findings:
Rate: Normal
Rhythm: Irregular
P wave: Each new p wave is different
PR interval: PR interval is variable (not constant)
QRS: Normal

Ectopic Beats:

PREMATURE ATRIAL CONTRACTION:

Single EKG strip

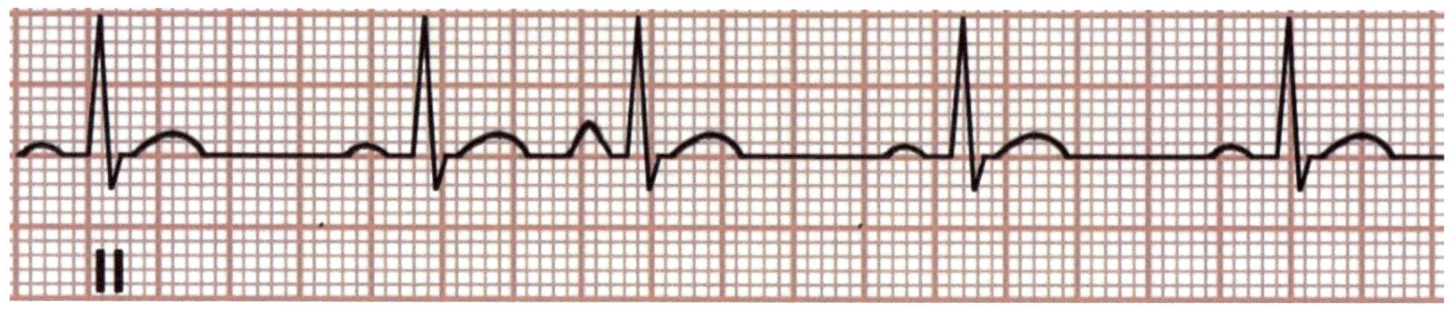

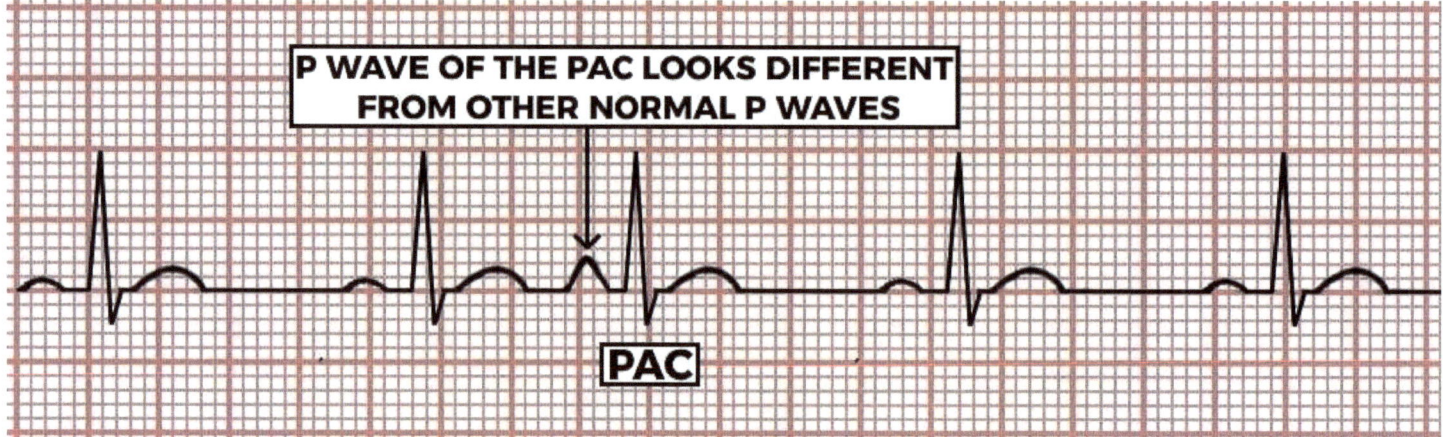

FIGURE 5 – 33: PREMATURE ATRIAL CONTRACTION

Etiology:
This is caused by a single automaticity focus located in the atria. This automaticity focus stimulates the atria to contract early outside the normal sinus routine controlled by the SA node. This contraction produces an abnormal-looking P wave that looks different compared to other P waves. This is because of the abnormal origin. This P wave also occurs earlier than the other P waves. The abnormal P wave is followed by a normal QRS complex and T wave. Hypoxia or electrolyte disorders can stimulate automaticity foci formation in the atrium.

EKG findings:
Rate: Normal rate
Rhythm: Irregular
P wave: The abnormal P wave looks different from other P waves.
PR interval: Normal
QRS: Normal

Clinical Features:
P Pulse: Normal rate + irregular
P Palpitation

Lab:
Best initial test: EKG

Treatment:
Reassurance

PREMATURE VENTRICULAR CONTRACTION:

Single EKG strip

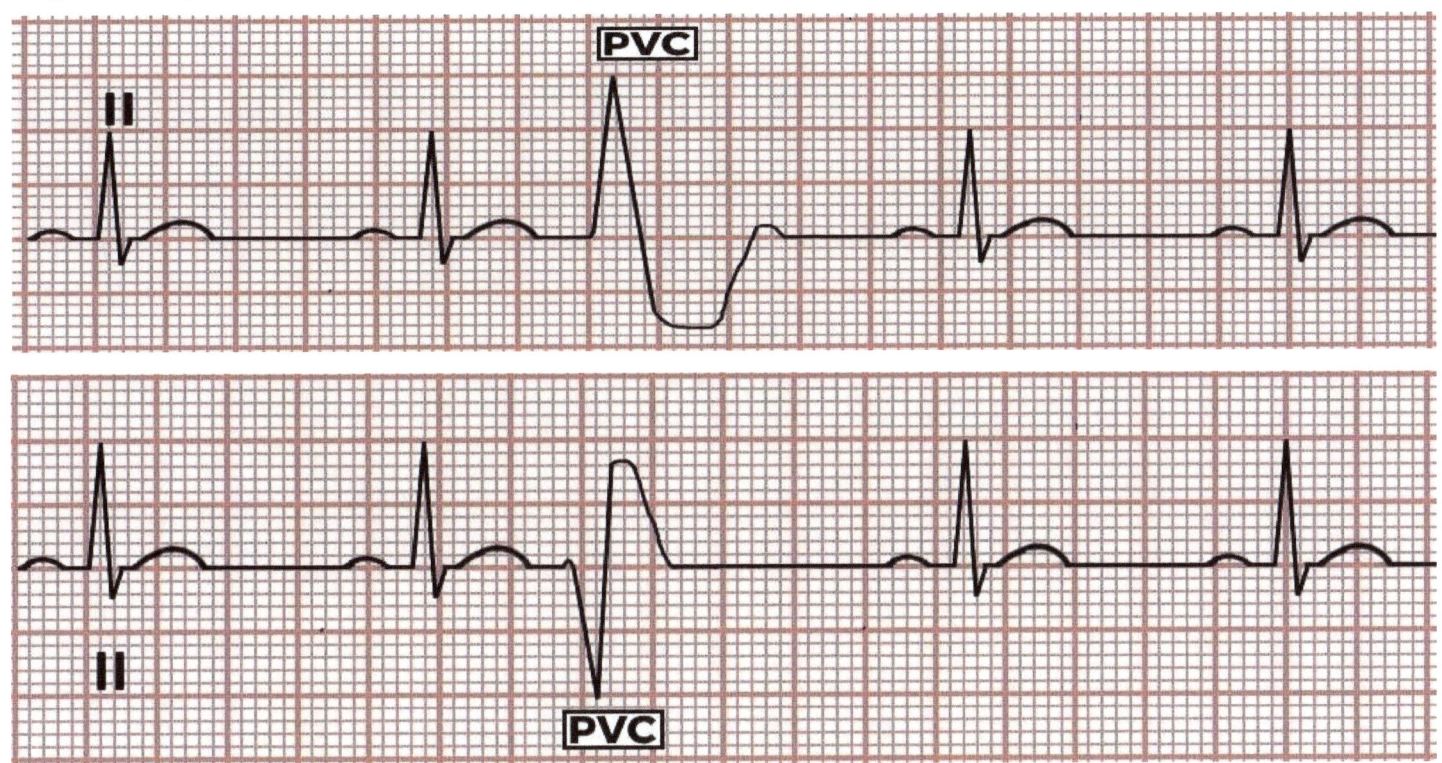

FIGURE 5 – 34: PREMATURE VENTRICULAR CONTRACTION

Etiology:
This is caused by a single automaticity focus located in the ventricle. This automaticity focus stimulates the ventricle to contract outside the normal sinus routine controlled by the SA node. This contraction produces a wide QRS complex. After the abnormal ventricular contraction, the normal rhythm resumes. The automaticity foci in the ventricle can be stimulated by hypoxia or electrolyte disorders.

EKG findings:
Rate: Normal rate
Rhythm: Irregular
P wave: Normal P wave
PR interval: Normal
QRS: Very tall and wide (greater than 120 ms)

Clinical Features:
P Pulse: Normal rate + irregular
P Palpitation

Lab:
Best initial test: EKG

Treatment:
Reassurance

Other EKG findings:

CONGENITAL LONG QT SYNDROME:

Single EKG strip:

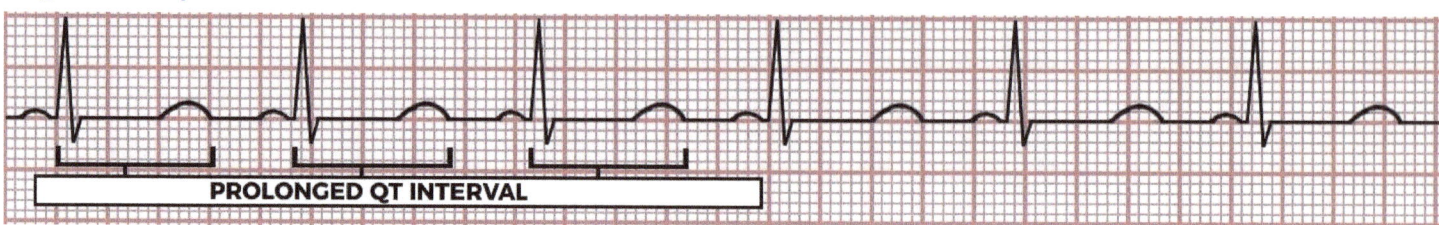

FIGURE 5 – 35: CONGENITAL LONG QT SYNDROME

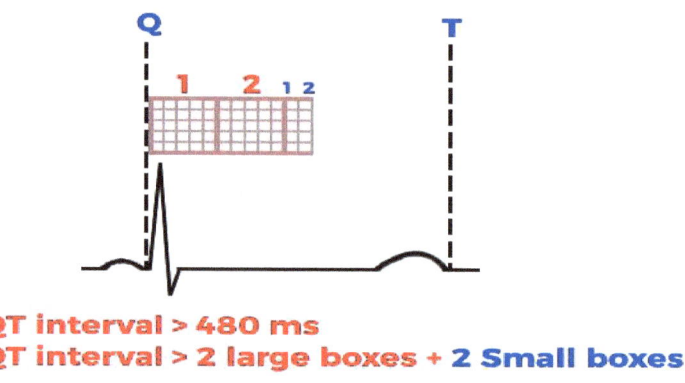

QT interval > 480 ms
QT interval > 2 large boxes + 2 Small boxes
Prolonged QT interval

ROMANO WARD SYNDROME:
Etiology:
Autosomal dominant

Clinical Features:
Prolonged QT interval on EKG
+
Positive family history of a family member who died suddenly of cardiac death below 50 years of age

JERVELL AND LANGE NIELSEN SYNDROME:
Etiology:
Autosomal recessive and due to a mutation in Na and K channels.

Clinical features:
Prolonged QT interval on EKG
+
Sensorineural deafness
Palpitation
Loss of consciousness

Lab:
Best initial test: EKG: Shows a Prolonged QT interval (Greater than 480 ms)

Treatment:
  A. **QT interval is prolonged + No syncope:**
     Propranolol

  B. **QT interval is prolonged + Syncope present:**
     Propranolol and Pacemaker

FIGURE 5 – 36: CONGENITAL LONG QT SYNDROME

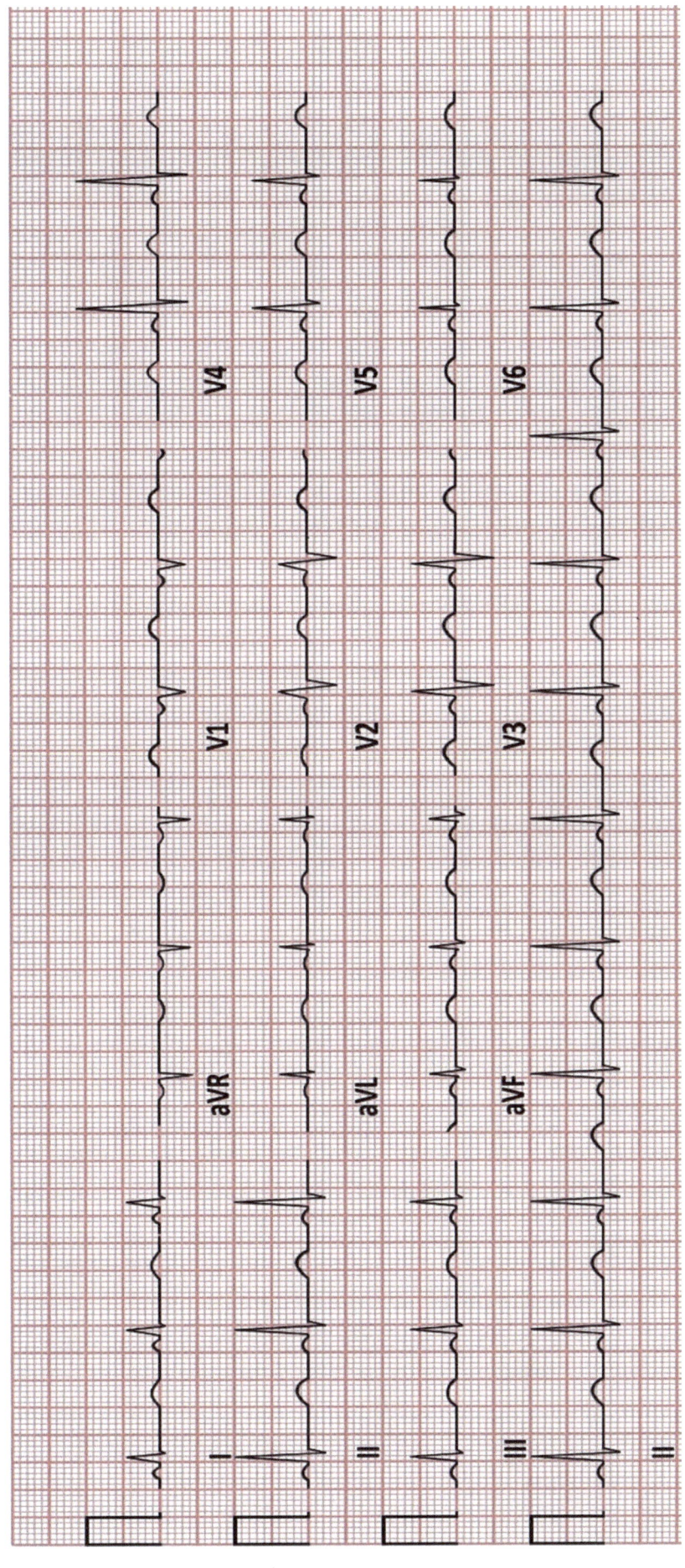

EKG Findings:
Rate: Normal
Rhythm: Regular
P wave: Normal
PR interval: Normal
QRS: Normal
+
QT interval is prolonged (Greater than 480ms)

HYPOTHERMIA

Single EKG strip:

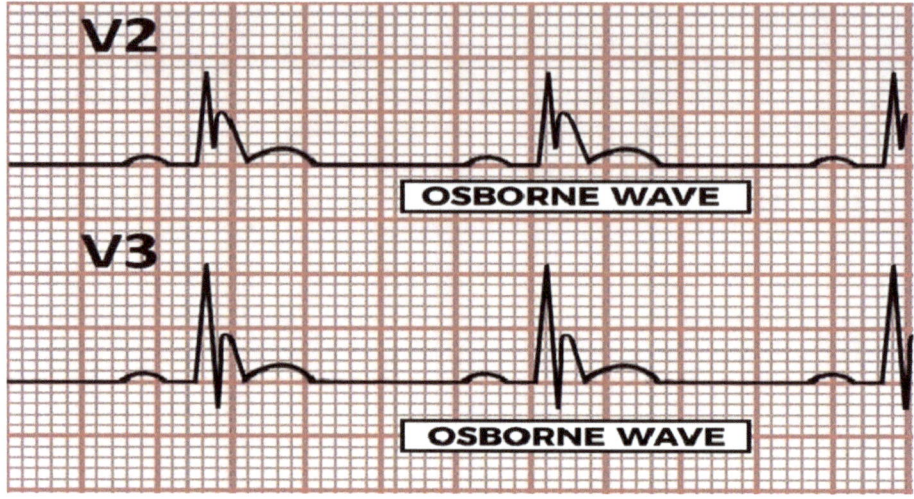

FIGURE 5 – 37: HYPOTHERMIA

Etiology:
This EKG pattern is caused by exposure to cold temperatures and is characterized by the appearance of an **Osborne wave or J wave.**

EKG:
Rate: Bradycardia
Rhythm: Regular
P wave: Normal
PR interval: Normal
QRS: Normal or wide + presence of **Osborne wave or J wave.**

Clinical features:
1. Mild hypothermia:
Temperature ranges between 32 – 35°C
Tachycardia
Tachypnea
+
Homeless or Alcoholic and found unconscious in the snow or cold

2. Moderate hypothermia:
Temperature ranges between 28 – 32°C
Bradycardia
+
Homeless or Alcoholic and found unconscious in the snow or cold

3. Severe Hypothermia:
Temperature is less than 28°C
Bradycardia
Coma
+
Homeless or Alcoholic and found unconscious in the snow or cold

Lab:
Best initial test: EKG

Treatment:
After the patient has warmed up, the EKG findings will return back to normal.

ELECTROLYTE DISORDERS

POTASSIUM	CALCIUM
Hypokalemia: **Etiology:** This is due to low potassium. Less than 3.5 mEq/L **EKG findings:** Flat T wave Prominent U wave 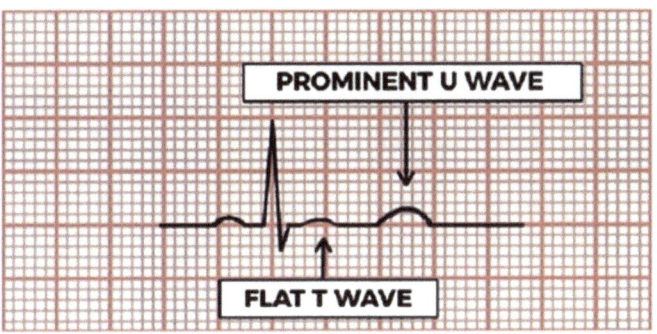	**Hypocalcemia:** **Etiology:** This is due to low calcium. Less than 8.5 mg/dL **EKG findings:** Prolonged QT interval > 480ms 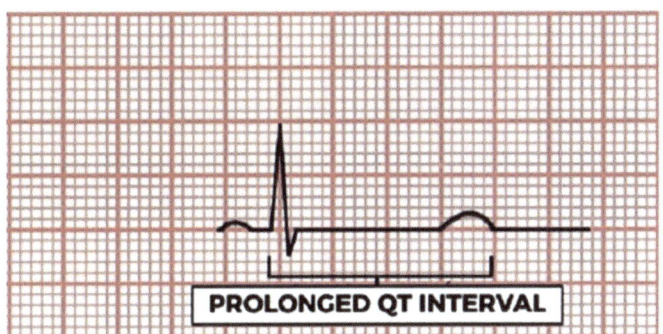
Hyperkalemia: **Etiology:** This is due to high potassium. Greater than 5.5 mEq/L **EKG findings:** P wave flattened Prolonged PR interval > 200ms QRS is wide > 120ms T wave is peaked 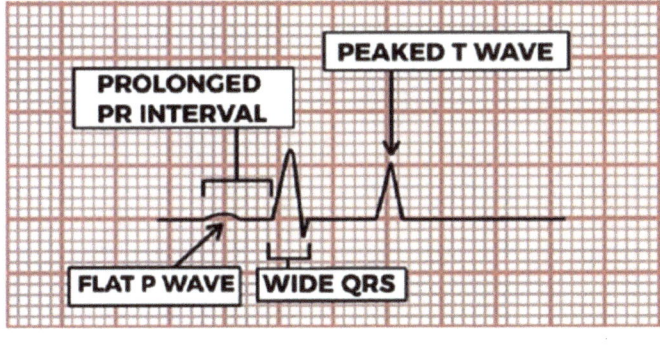	**Hypercalcemia:** **Etiology:** This is due to high calcium. Greater than 10.5 mg/dL **EKG findings:** Shortened QT interval less than 360ms 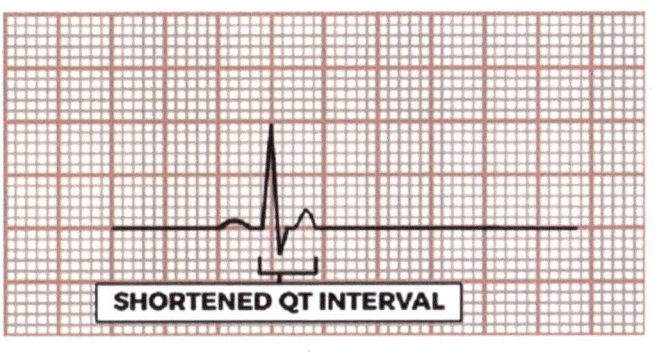

ASYSTOLE

Single EKG strip:

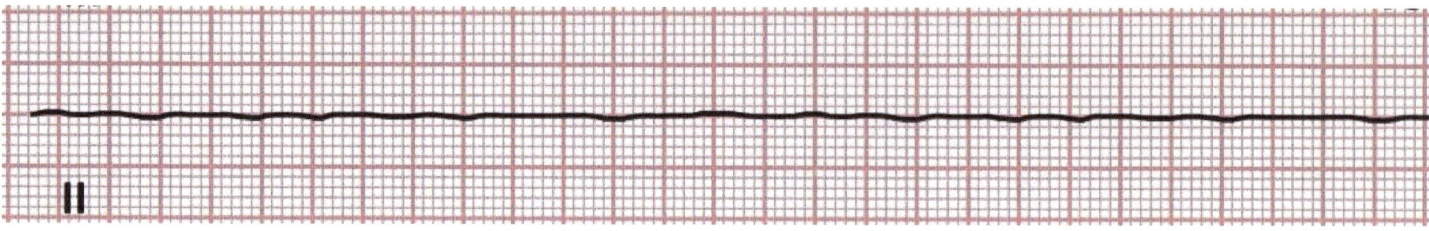

FIGURE 5 – 38: ASYSTOLE

Etiology:
No electrical activity in the heart
+
No mechanical contraction of the heart

Clinical features: PUB
P Pulseless
U Unconscious
B BP Low (Hypotensive)

EKG findings:
It looks like a straight horizontal line on the EKG
Rate: No rate
Rhythm: No rhythm
P wave: None
PR interval: None
QRS: None

Treatment:
Follow the ACLS flow chart

ACLS flow chart:

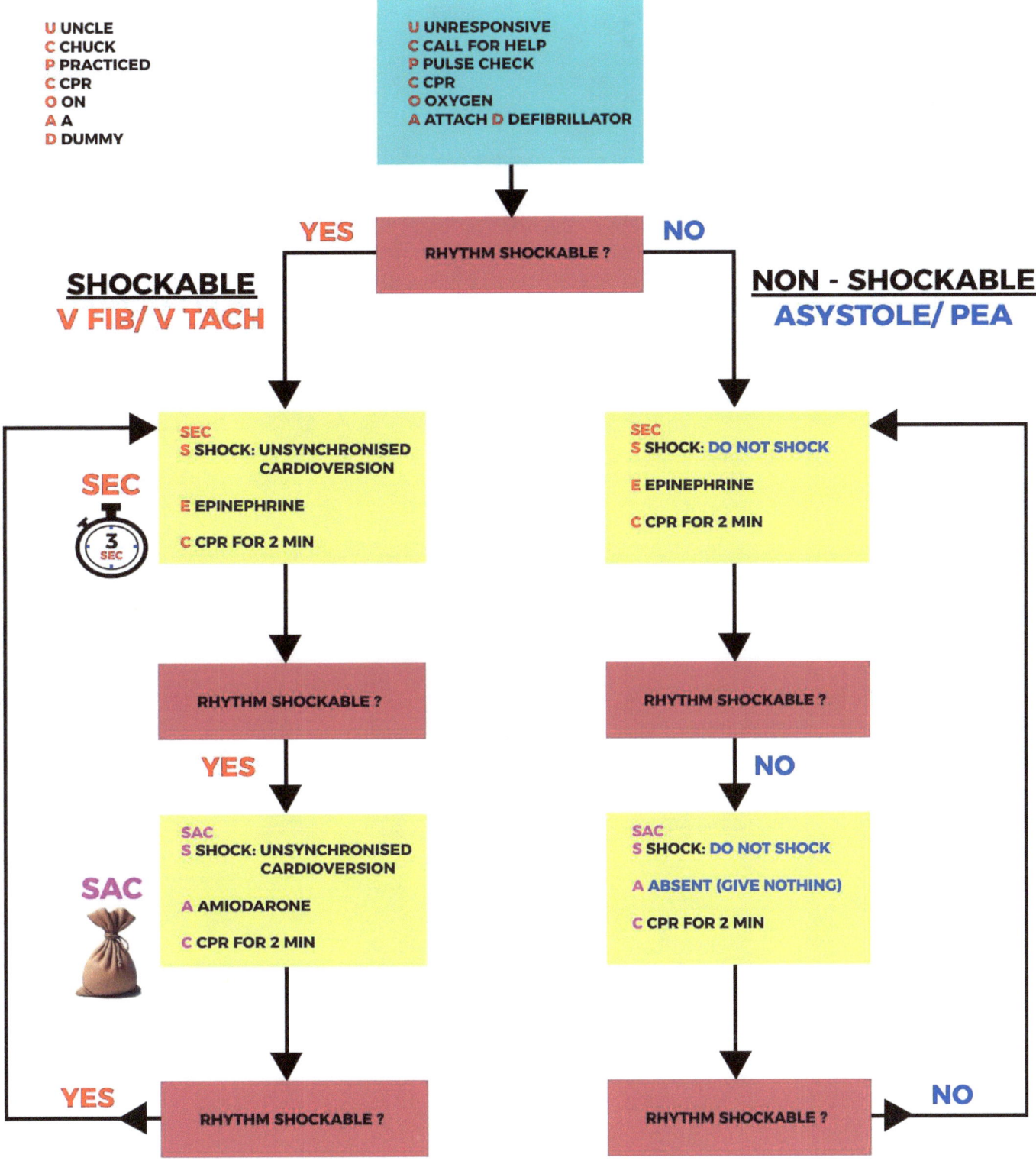

FIGURE 5 – 39: ACLS TREATMENT FLOWCHART FOR ASYSTOLE

PULSELESS ELECTRICAL ACTIVITY:

Etiology:
The heart's electrical activity is **present**
+
No mechanical contraction of the heart

Cause:
5 H and 5T

5 H	5 T
H Hypovole**mia**	**T** Tension Pneumothorax
H Hyperther**mia**	**T** Tamponade (Cardiac tamponade)
H Hypokale**mia**	**T** Thrombus (Pulmonary embolism)
H Hypoxe**mia**	**T** Trauma
H Hydrogen ion (Acidosis)	**T** Toxins

EKG findings:
Rate: Normal rate
Rhythm: Regular rhythm
P wave: Normal P wave
PR interval: Normal PR interval
QRS: Normal QRS

Clinical Features:
Normal sinus rhythm on EKG
+
PUB
P Pulseless
U Unconscious
B BP Low (Hypotensive)

Treatment:
Treat the underlying cause and follow the ACLS flowchart.

ACLS flow chart:

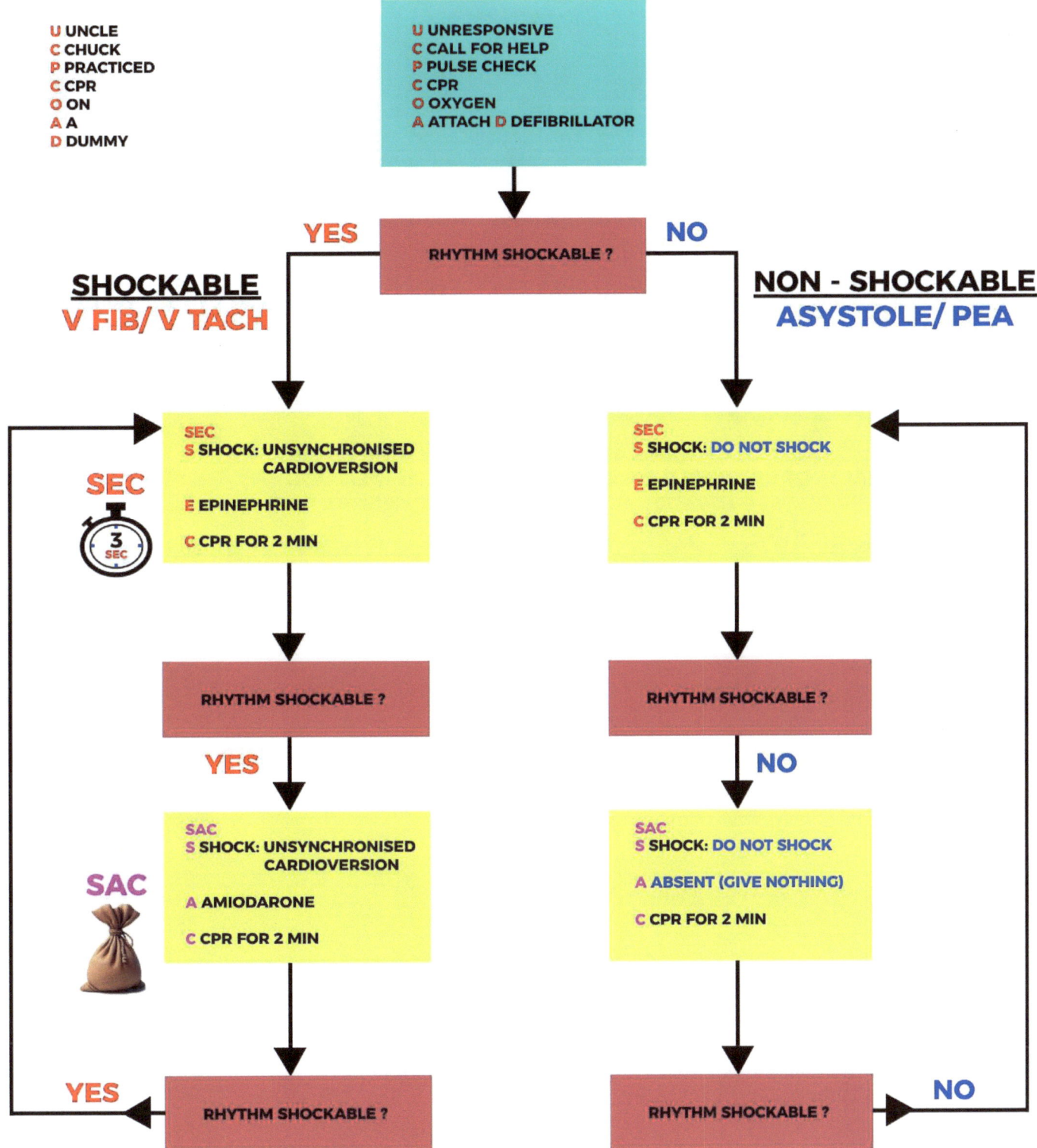

FIGURE 5 – 40: ACLS TREATMENT FLOWCHART FOR PULSELESS ELECTRICAL ACTIVITY(PEA)

ELECTRICAL ALTERNANS IN PERICARDIAL EFFUSION:

Single EKG strip:

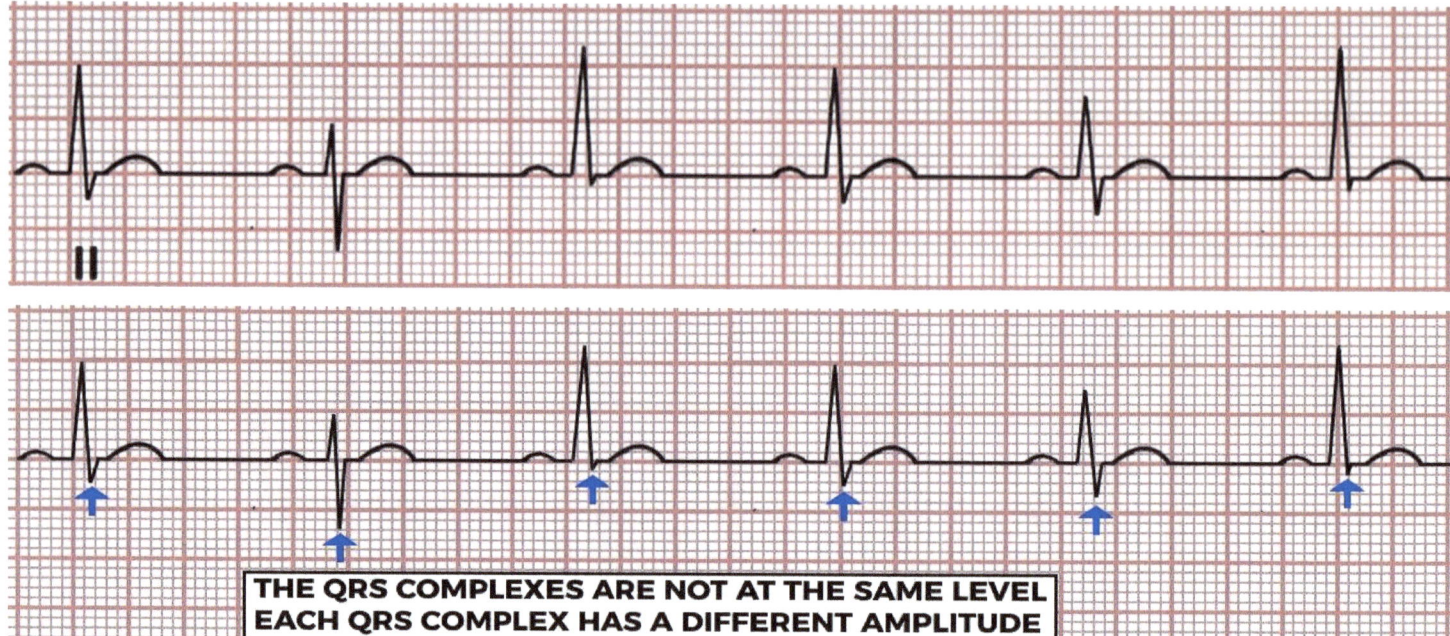

FIGURE 5 – 41: ELECTRICAL ALTERNANS

Etiology:
The movement of fluid within the pericardium causes a unique EKG pattern, with each QRS varying in amplitude (height).

Cause:
Pericardial effusion

EKG findings:
Rate: Normal
Rhythm: Regular
P wave: Normal
PR interval: Normal
QRS: The QRS complexes have varying amplitude (height)

Clinical features: HDDPPP
H Hypotension
D Distended neck veins
D Distant heart sound (or Muffled Heart sound)
P Pulse rate increased (Tachycardia)
P Pulsus paradoxus (inspiration causes a decrease in systolic BP > 10 mmHg)
P PMI (Point of Maximal Impulse) is not palpable.

Lab:
Best initial test: Echocardiogram
EKG: Shows Electrical alternans
Chest X-ray: Shows a globular Heart or Water bottle shaped heart

Treatment:
Best initial treatment: IV Fluids to increase the blood pressure
Definitive treatment: Pericardiocentesis

FIGURE 5-42: ELECTRICAL ALTERNANS

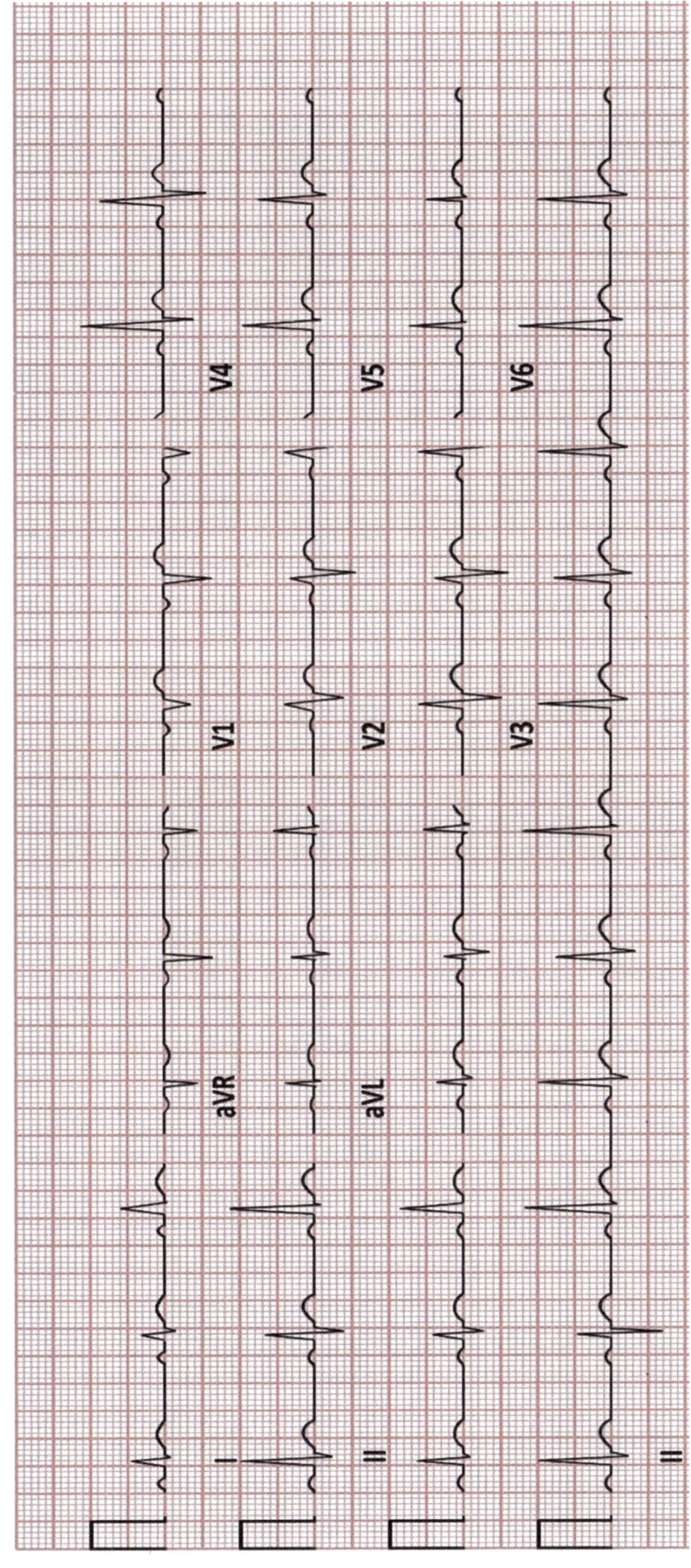

EKG findings:
Rate: Normal
Rhythm: Regular
P wave: Normal
PR interval: Normal
QRS: Each QRS has varying amplitude (height)

PULMONARY EMBOLISM:

Single EKG strip:

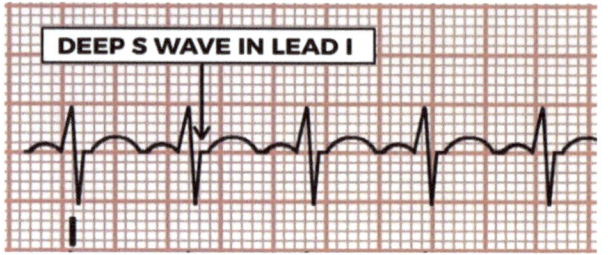 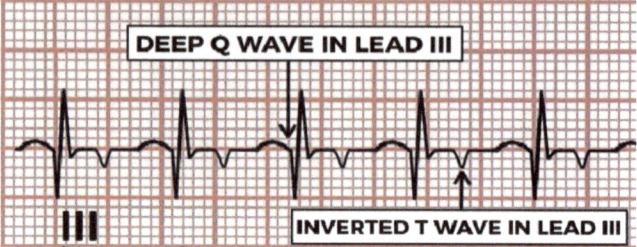

FIGURE 5 – 43: PULMONARY EMBOLISM

Etiology:
This is due to the obstruction of blood flow in the pulmonary artery by an emboli. This obstruction prevents the adequate oxygenation of blood leading to hypoxia.

EKG findings:
Rate: Tachycardia
Rhythm: Regular
P wave: Normal
PR interval: Normal
QRS: Normal
+

S1Q3T3 pattern:
1. Deep S wave in lead I
2. Deep Q wave in lead III
3. Inverted T wave in lead III

Clinical features:
Sudden onset of shortness of breath
Cough
Chest pain (Pleuritic: worse on inspiration)
Hemoptysis
+
Tachycardia
Tachypnea
Hypotension
Chest is clear on auscultation
+
History of **DISC:**
D Deep Venous Thrombosis (DVT)
I Immobilization
S Surgery
C Contraceptive use
C Cancer

Lab:
Most accurate test: Pulmonary CT Angiography

Treatment:
Treatment of Pulmonary embolism is dependent on various criteria and is beyond the scope of this book

FIGURE 5 – 44: PULMONARY EMBOLISM

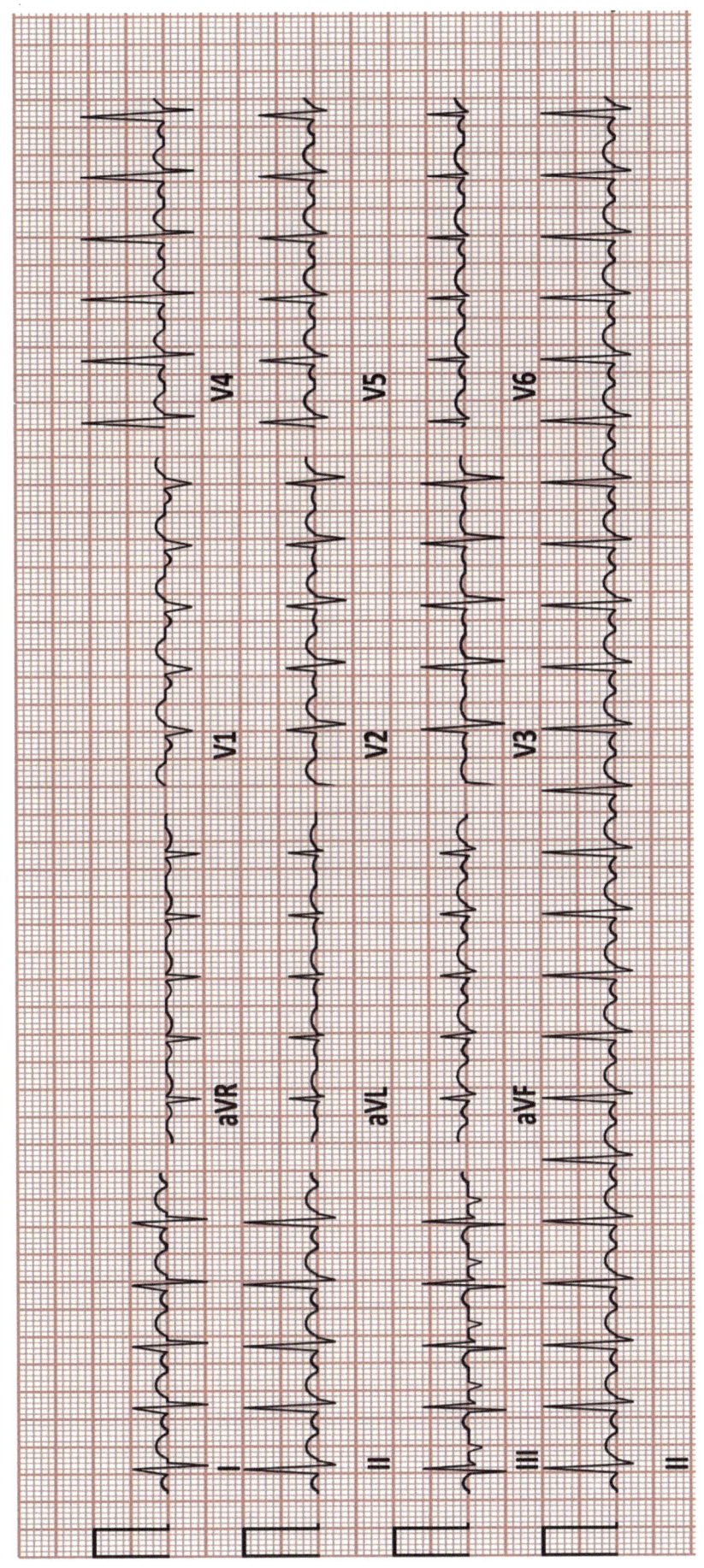

Rate: Tachycardia
Rhythm: Regular
P wave: Normal
PR interval: Normal
QRS: Normal
+
S1Q3T3 pattern: Deep S wave in lead I, Deep Q wave in lead III and Inverted T wave in lead III

ST ELEVATION/ DEPRESSION:

To understand the lead changes following myocardial ischemia or infarction, it is essential first to comprehend the blood supply to the heart.

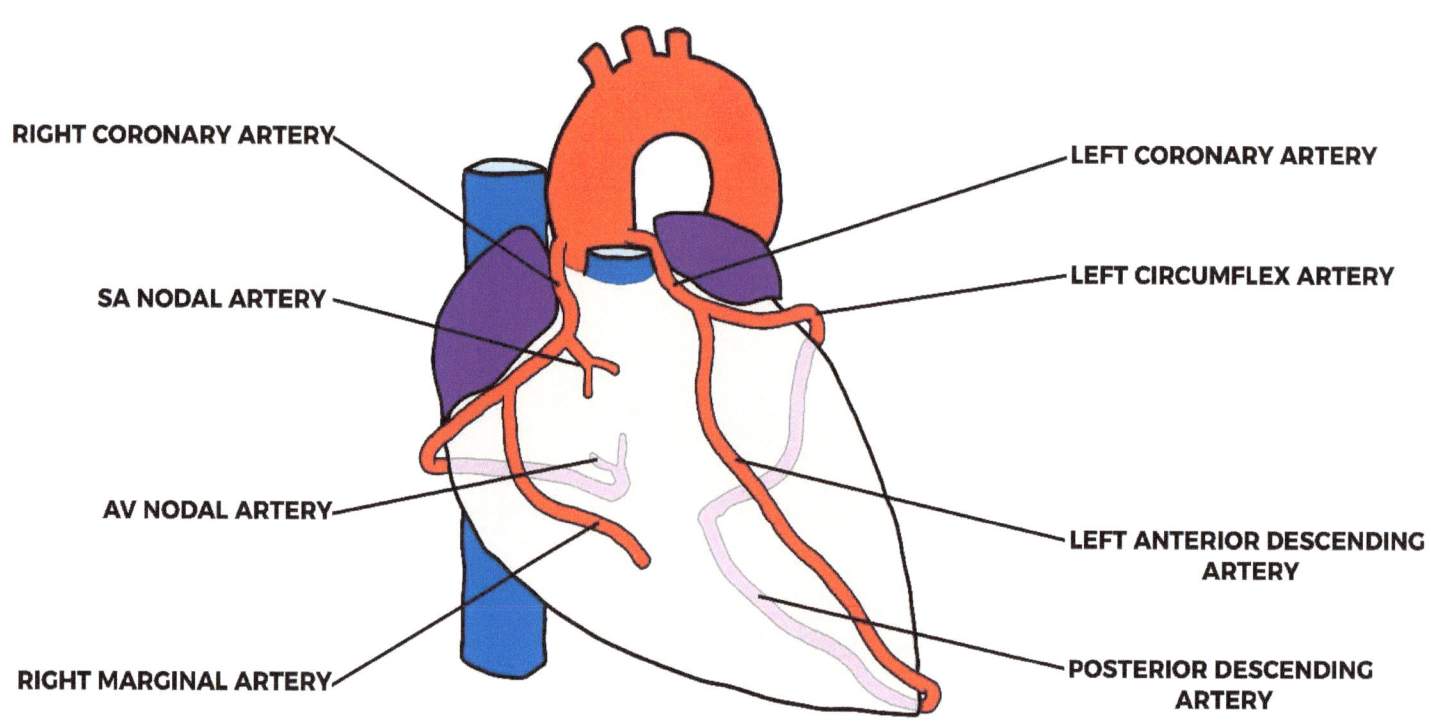

FIGURE 5 – 45: BLOOD SUPPLY TO THE HEART

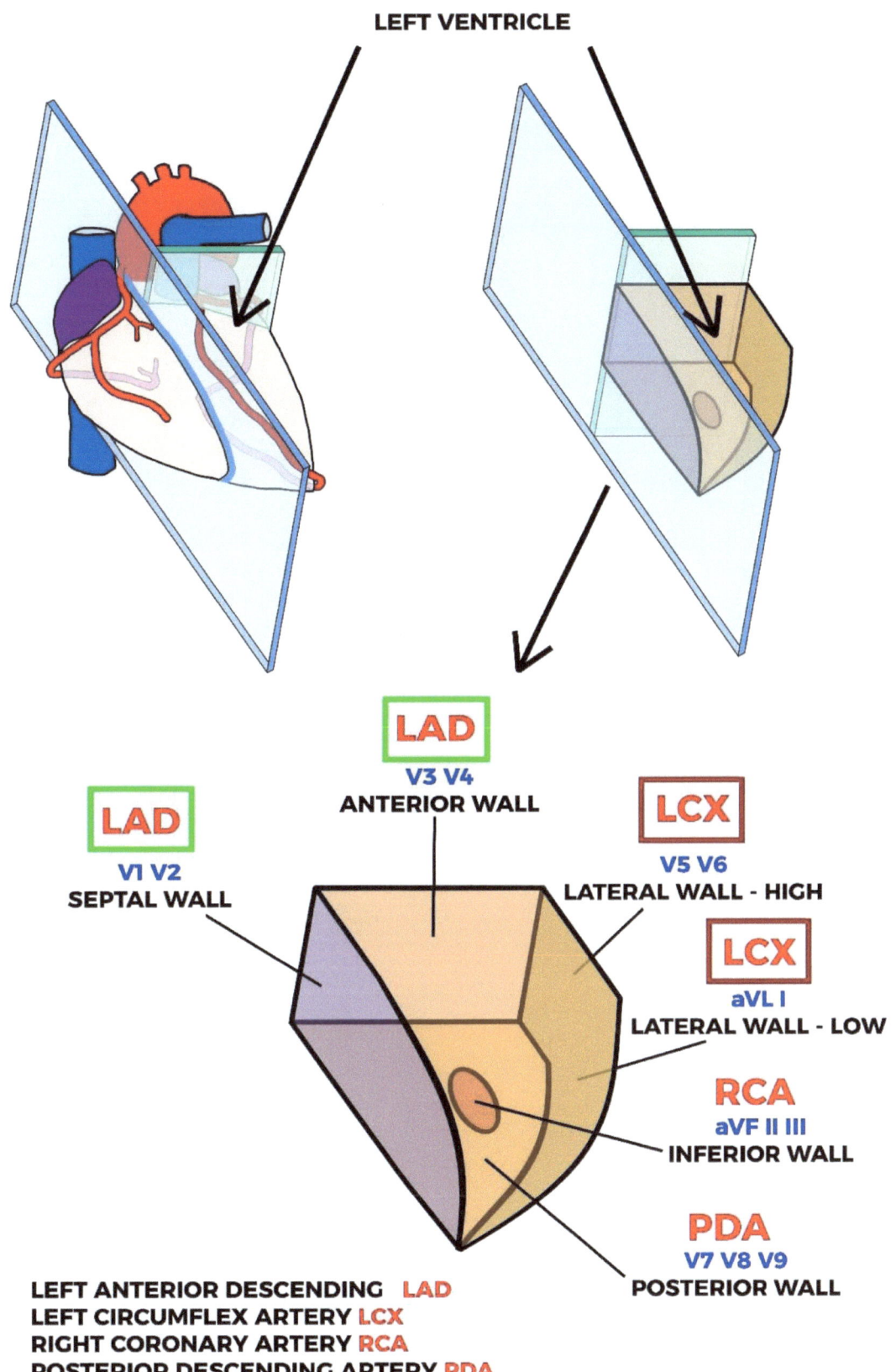

FIGURE 5 – 46: 3 – DIMENSIONAL IMAGE OF THE LEFT VENTRICLE TO SHOW THE LEADS INVOLVED FOLLOWING MYOCARDIAL ISCHEMIA OR INFARCTION (MARKS MODEL)

LOCATION OF MYOCARDIAL INFARCTION	LEADS WITH ST ELEVATION/ DEPRESSION	CORRESPONDING ARTERY AFFECTED
Septal	V1, V2	LEFT ANTERIOR DESCENDING ARTERY
Anterior	V3, V4	LEFT ANTERIOR DESCENDING ARTERY
Lateral	V5, V6	LEFT CIRCUMFLEX ARTERY
Lateral	I, aVL,	LEFT CIRCUMFLEX ARTERY
Inferior	II, III, aVF	RIGHT CORONARY ARTERY
Posterior	V7, V8, V9	POSTERIOR DESCENDING ARTERY

Question 11:
A 72-year-old woman complained of central chest pain radiating to her left arm. An EKG done showed ST elevation in lead V1 and V2. Which artery is likely affected?
   A. Left anterior descending artery
   B. Left circumflex artery
   C. Posterior descending artery
   D. Right marginal artery

Question 11 Answer: A. Left anterior descending artery. ST elevation in lead V1 and V2 indicates this patient has a septal infarct. The artery that supplies the septal region is the left anterior descending artery.

ST DEPRESSION

Single EKG strip:

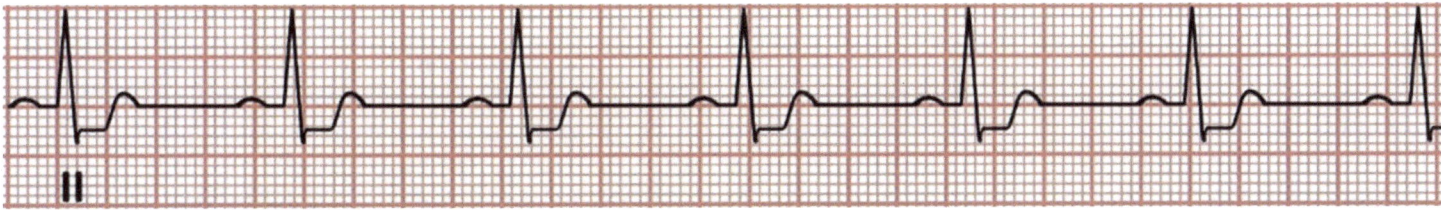

FIGURE 5 –47: ST DEPRESSION

Diagram:

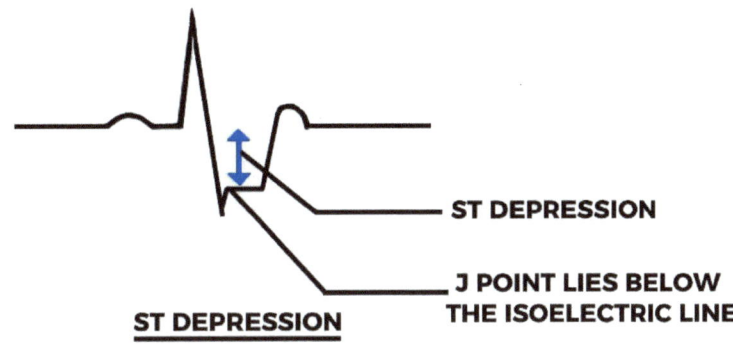

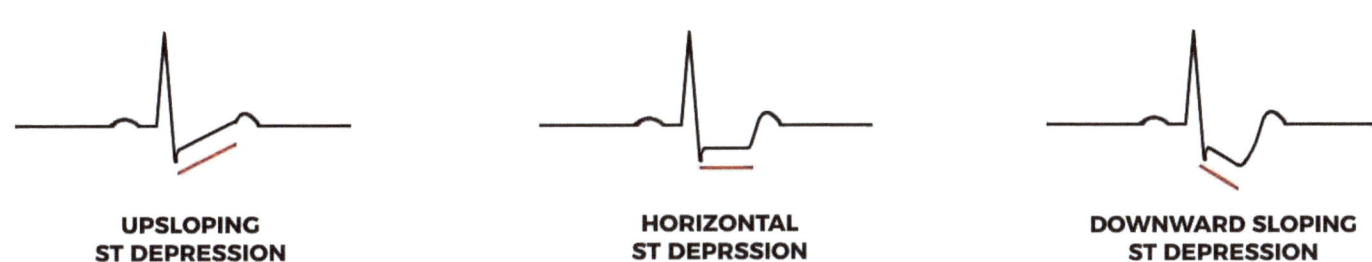

Etiology:

ST depression is a finding seen on an EKG and is due to Stable Angina, Unstable Angina, or Non-ST Elevated Myocardial Infarction (NSTEMI). ST depression occurs when the J point lies below the isoelectric line in 2 or more contiguous leads. The J point is the point where the end of the QRS complex meets the beginning of the ST segment.

STABLE ANGINA	UNSTABLE ANGINA	NON-ST ELEVATED MYOCARDIAL INFARCTION (NSTEMI)
Etiology: Atherosclerosis of the coronary artery ↓ **> 70%** of coronary artery **blocked** (No Acute Atherosclerosis Rupture) No ischemia or infarction **Normal** Troponin and CKMB	Etiology: Acute Atherosclerosis Rupture ↓ Thrombose formation ↓ **> 90%** of coronary artery **blocked** ↓ Sub endocardial ischemia + **Normal** Troponin and CKMB	Etiology: Acute Atherosclerosis Rupture ↓ Thrombose formation ↓ **> 90%** of coronary artery **blocked** ↓ Sub endocardial Infarction + **Elevated** Troponin and CKMB

STABLE ANGINA	UNSTABLE ANGINA	NON-ST ELEVATED MYOCARDIAL INFARCTION (NSTEMI)
Clinical features: Chest pain: 　**Location:** Substernal 　**Radiating:** To the Left arm 　**Duration:** Less than 20 min 　**Aggravated:** Only after exercise 　**Relieved:** Relieved by rest and Nitroglycerine + **T** Tightness of the chest **S** Sweating **S** Shortness of breath **N** Nausea and vomiting	**Clinical features:** Chest pain: 　**Location:** Substernal 　**Radiating:** To the Left arm 　**Duration:** Greater than 20 min 　**Aggravated:** None, starts suddenly 　**Relieved:** Not relieved by rest or Nitroglycerine + **T** Tightness of the chest **S** Sweating **S** Shortness of breath **N** Nausea and vomiting	**Clinical features:** Chest pain: 　**Location:** Substernal 　**Radiating:** To the Left arm 　**Duration:** Greater than 20 min 　**Aggravated:** None, starts suddenly 　**Relieved:** Not relieved by rest or Nitroglycerine + **T** Tightness of the chest **S** Sweating **S** Shortness of breath **N** Nausea and vomiting
Lab: **Best initial test:** EKG: shows ST depression or a normal EKG ↓ **Next best test:** Troponin: Normal Troponin and CKMB + History of Chest pain relieved by rest. ↓ **Stress test:** Positive stress test (ST depression >2 mm following exercise)	**Lab:** **Best initial test:** EKG: shows ST depression or a normal EKG ↓ **Next best test:** Troponin: Normal Troponin and CKMB + History of Chest pain NOT relieved by rest ↓ **Coronary Catheterization**	**Lab:** **Best initial test:** EKG: shows ST depression or a normal EKG ↓ **Next best test:** Troponin: Elevated Troponin and CKMB (once the Troponin level is elevated, you do not need a history of chest pain to proceed to coronary catheterization) ↓ **Coronary Catheterization:**
Treatment: Elective Coronary Catheterization and Stent placement + **(BLA NITRATES)** **B** Blood pressure control: 　1. BB (Beta Blockers) 　2. ACE I (Angiotensin Converting Enzyme Inhibitors) **L** Lipids: 　Statins: Atorvastatin **A** Antiplatelet 　Aspirin: (**Decreases mortality**) 　　+ 　Clopidogrel (P2Y12 inhibitor) + **Nitrates (Long-acting)**	**Treatment:** **Definitive treatment** Stent: Done if 2 arteries are affected CABG: Done if 3 or more arteries are affected **Supportive treatment: MONAA** **M** Morphine **O** Oxygen **N** Nitrate **A** Antiplatelet Aspirin **A** Anticoagulant: Heparin **Discharge Home on:** **(BLA No NITRATES)** **B** Blood pressure: BB, ACE I **L** Lipid: Statins: Atorvastatin **A** Antiplatelet: Aspirin + Clopidogrel + **No Nitrates**	**Treatment:** **Definitive treatment** Stent: Done if 2 arteries are affected CABG: Done if 3 or more arteries are affected **Supportive treatment: MONAA** **M** Morphine **O** Oxygen **N** Nitrate **A** Antiplatelet Aspirin **A** Anticoagulant: Heparin **Discharge Home on:** **(BLA No NITRATES)** **B** Blood pressure: BB, ACE I **L** Lipid: Statins: Atorvastatin **A** Antiplatelet: Aspirin + Clopidogrel + **No Nitrates**

FIGURE 5 – 48: ST DEPRESSION

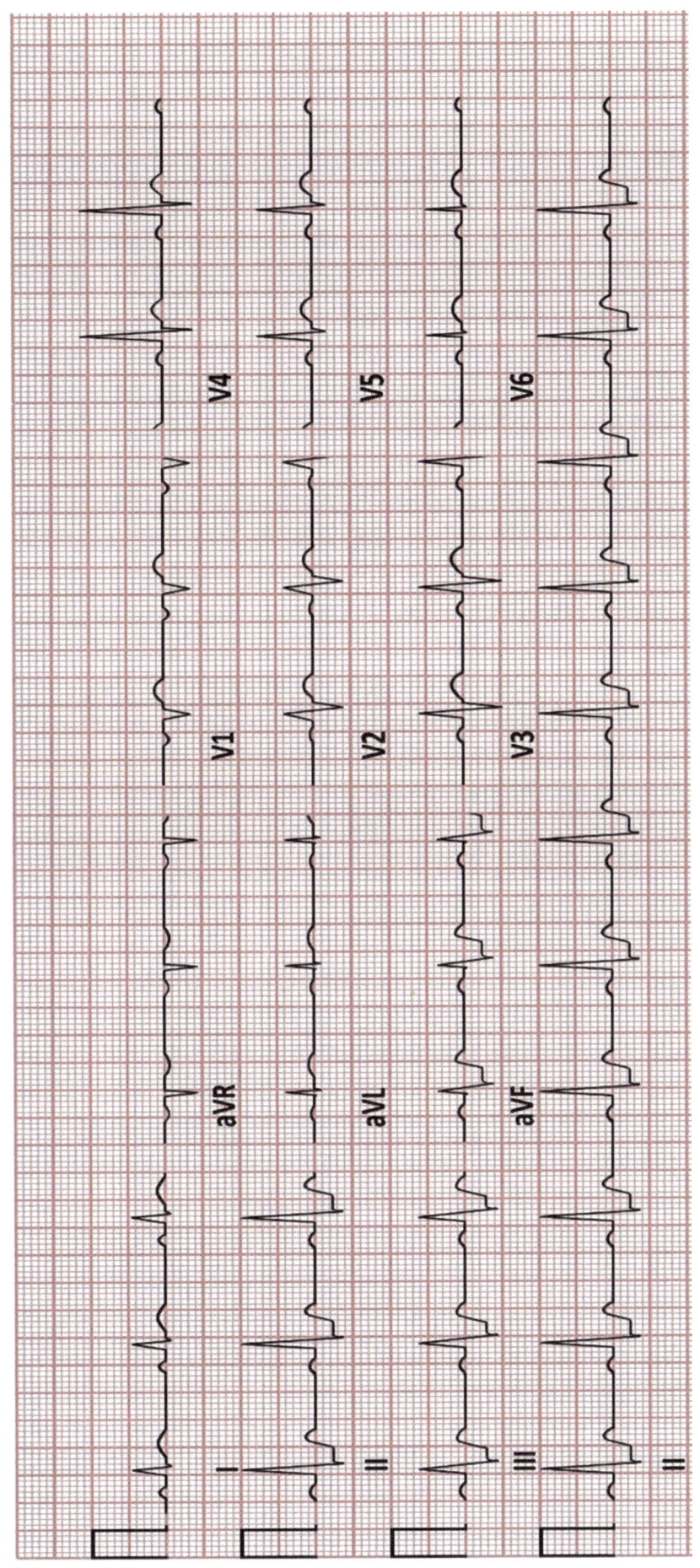

EKG Findings:
Rate: Normal
Rhythm: Regular
P wave: Normal
PR interval: Normal
QRS: Normal
+
ST depression in Lead II, III and aVF

ST ELEVATION

Single EKG strip:

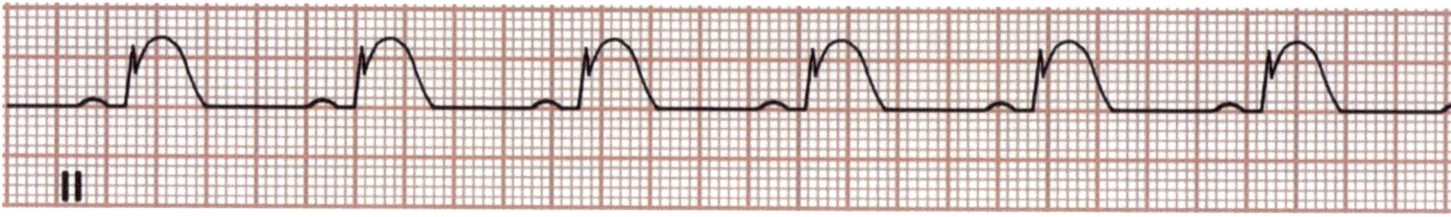

FIGURE 5 – 49: ST ELEVATION

Diagram:

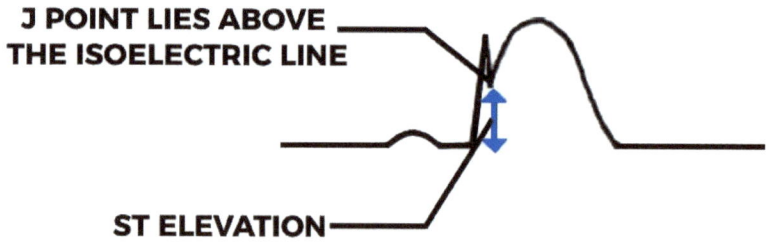

ST ELEVATION

Etiology:
ST elevation is a finding seen on an EKG following ST Elevation Myocardial Infarction (STEMI). ST elevation occurs when the J point lies above the isoelectric line in 2 or more contiguous leads. The J point is the point where the QRS complex meets the ST segment. ST elevation is measured from the isoelectric line to the j point. ST elevation is when there is an elevation greater than 2mm in V1 – V6 and 1 mm in other leads.

> Acute Atherosclerosis Rupture
> ↓
> Thrombose formation
> ↓
> **100%** of coronary artery **blocked**
> ↓
> Transmural **Infarction** (infarction of the entire thickness of the myocardium)
> +
> **Elevated** Troponin and CKMB

Clinical features:
Chest pain:
   Location: Substernal
   Radiating: To the Left arm, neck, or jaw
   Duration: Greater than 20 min
   Aggravated: No Aggravating factors prior to onset of chest pain. Chest pain starts suddenly.
   Relieved: Not relieved by rest or Nitroglycerine
+
T Tightness of the chest
S Sweating
S Shortness of breath
N Nausea and vomiting

Lab:
Best initial test: EKG shows ST **Elevation**
↓
Next best test: Troponin: **Elevated** Troponin and CKMB
↓
Coronary Catheterization

Treatment:
Definitive treatment
Stent Placement: Done if 2 or less Coronary arteries are affected
Coronary Artery Bypass Grafting (CABG): Done if 3 or more coronary arteries are affected

Supportive treatment: MONA
M Morphine
O Oxygen
N Nitrate
A Antiplatelet Aspirin
A Anticoagulant: Heparin

Discharge Home on:
(BLA No NITRATES)
B Blood Pressure control: Beta Blocker, ACE Inhibitor
L Lipid: Statin: Atorvastatin
A Aspirin + Clopidogrel
+
No Nitrates

FIGURE 5 – 50: ST ELEVATION

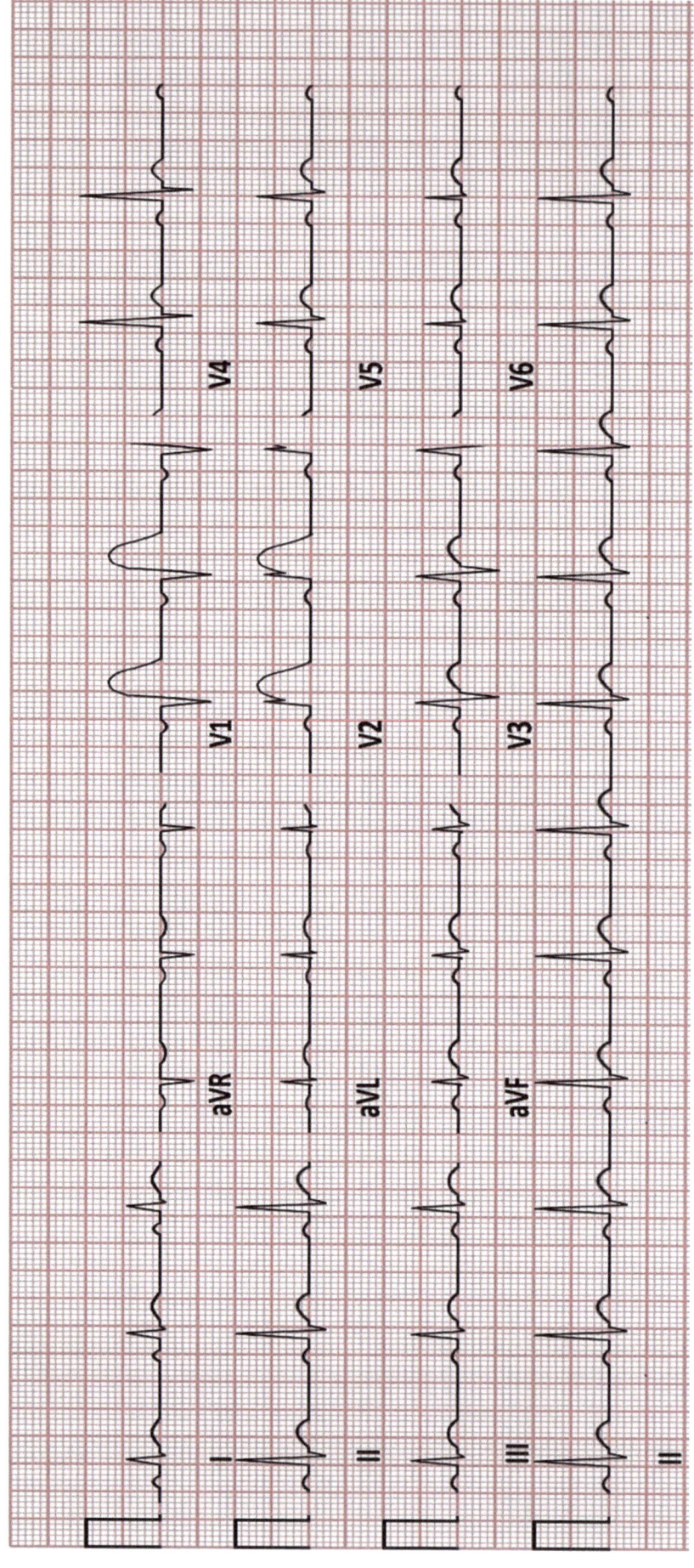

EKG Findings:
Rate: Normal
Rhythm: Regular
P wave: Normal
PR interval: Normal
QRS: Normal
+
ST elevation in Lead V1 and V2

Question 12:
A 69-year-old male suddenly complained of central chest pain radiating to his jaw while watching television. An EKG done showed ST elevation in lead I and aVL. Which artery is likely affected?
- A. Left anterior descending artery
- B. Left circumflex artery
- C. Posterior descending artery
- D. Right marginal artery

Question 12 Answer: B. Left circumflex artery. ST elevation in lead I and aVL indicates this patient has a lateral infarct. The artery that supplies the lateral region is the left circumflex artery.

ST ELEVATION WITH RECIPROCAL ST DEPRESSION:

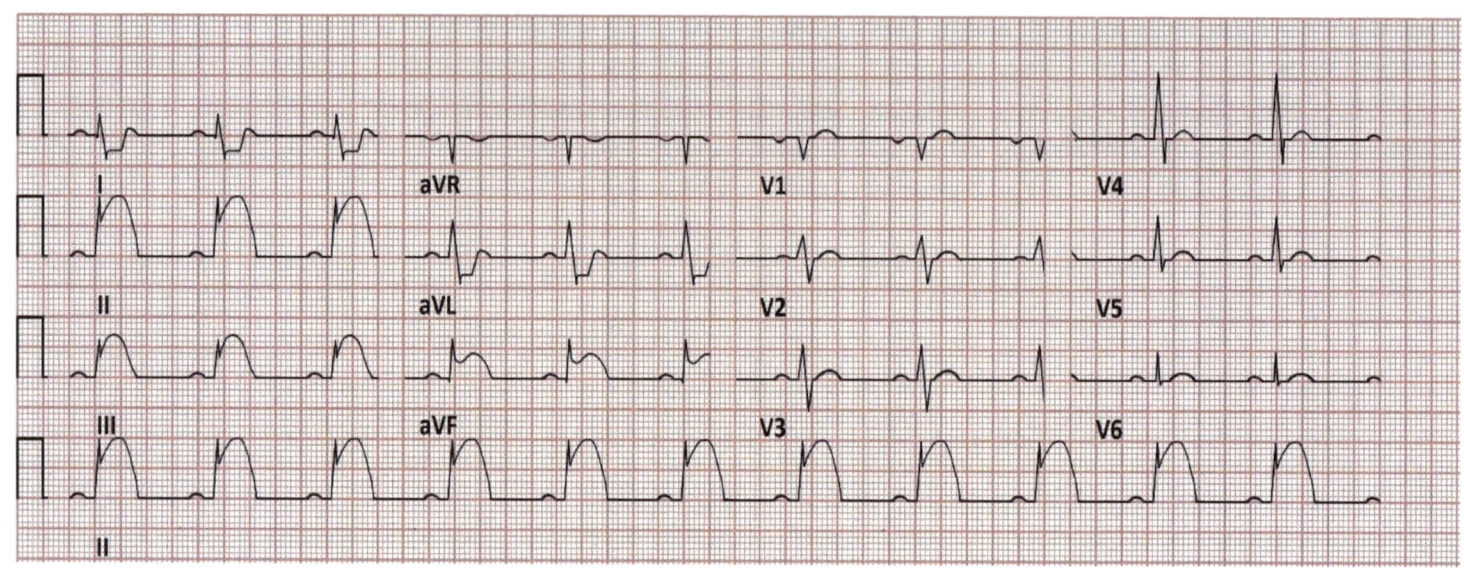

FIGURE 5 – 51: ST ELEVATION WITH RECIPROCAL ST DEPRESSION

The above EKG is one you definitely need to know. It shows the ST elevation in lead II, III, and aVF with reciprocal ST depression in I and aVL. Two sets of leads in particular that mirror themselves are II, III, and aVF, and I and aVL. So when there is myocardial infarction involving **the right coronary artery**, there will be ST elevation on II, III, and aVF and reciprocal ST depression on I and aVL. When there is myocardial infarction involving **the left circumflex artery**, there will be ST elevation on I and aVL and reciprocal ST depression on II, III, and aVF. There is nothing like ST depression with reciprocal ST elevation. Once you see ST elevation mixed with ST depression in an EKG, the diagnosis is Myocardial infarction and never myocardial ischemia or pericarditis.

LOCATION OF MYOCARDIAL INFARCTION	LEADS WITH ST ELEVATION	LEADS WITH RECIPROCAL ST DEPRESSION
Septal	V1, V2	V7, V8, V9
Anterior	V3, V4	None
Lateral	I, aVL, V5, V6	II, III, aVF
Inferior	II, III, aVF	I, aVL
Posterior	V7, V8, V9	V1, V2

FIGURE 5-52: ST ELEVATION WITH RECIPROCAL ST DEPRESSION

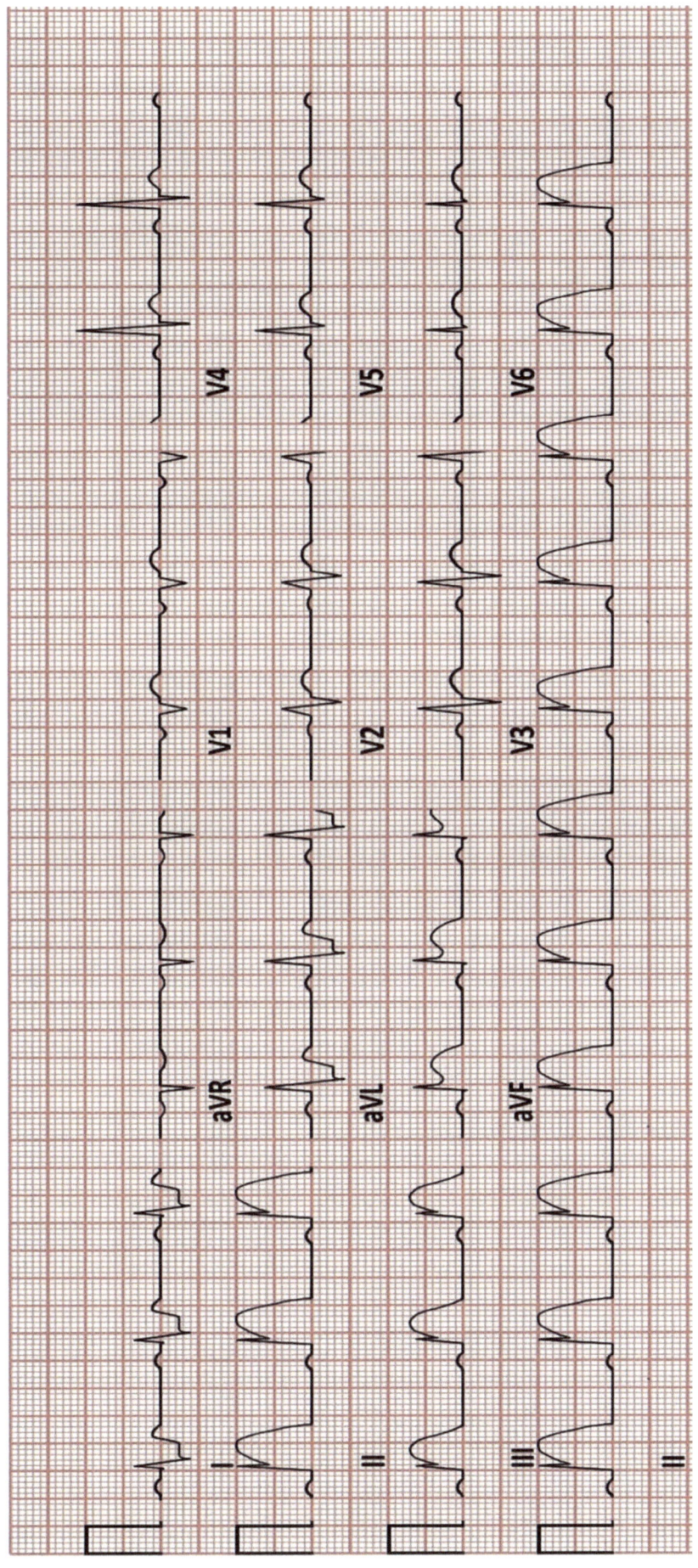

EKG Findings:
Rate: Normal
Rhythm: Regular
P wave: Normal
PR interval: Normal
QRS: Normal
+
ST elevation in Lead II, III and aVF + reciprocal ST depression I and aVL

ST ELEVATION IN PERICARDITIS

Diagram:

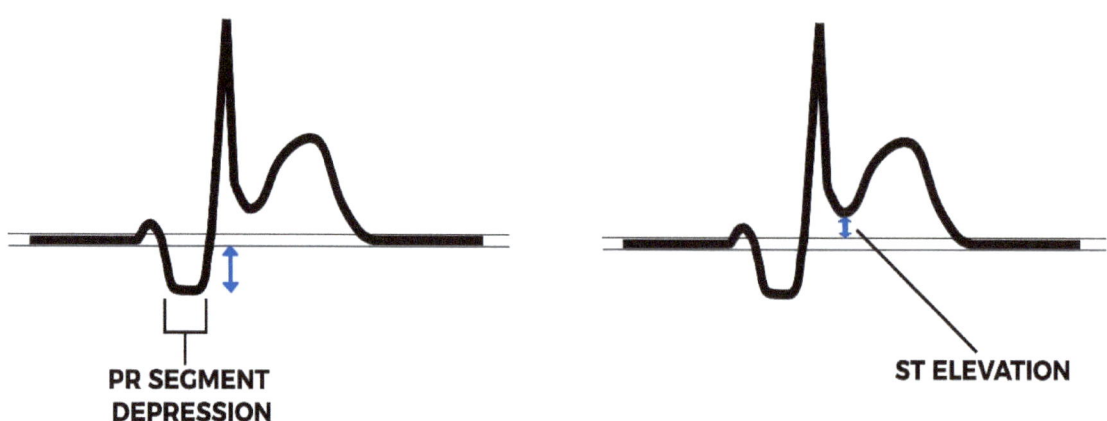

Etiology:
Pericarditis is the inflammation of the pericardium of the heart. In pericarditis, there is widespread ST elevation and PR segment depression, which is a very unique EKG presentation.

Clinical features: CAR UP
Upper respiratory tract infection (URTI) 2 weeks earlier
↓
C Chest pain
A Aggravated: Inspiration, lying flat
R Relieved: Leaning forward, sitting up
U URTI recent
P Pericardial friction Rub (Squeaking sound)
P Pulsus paradoxus (inspiration causes a decrease in systolic BP > 10 mmHg)

Lab:
Best initial test: ECG: Shows widespread ST elevation (diffuse ST elevation) and PR segment depression

Treatment:
1st line NSAID
OR
2nd line Colchicine
Avoid STEROIDS. The option with steroids is always wrong.

FIGURE 5-53: ST ELEVATION IN PERICARDITIS

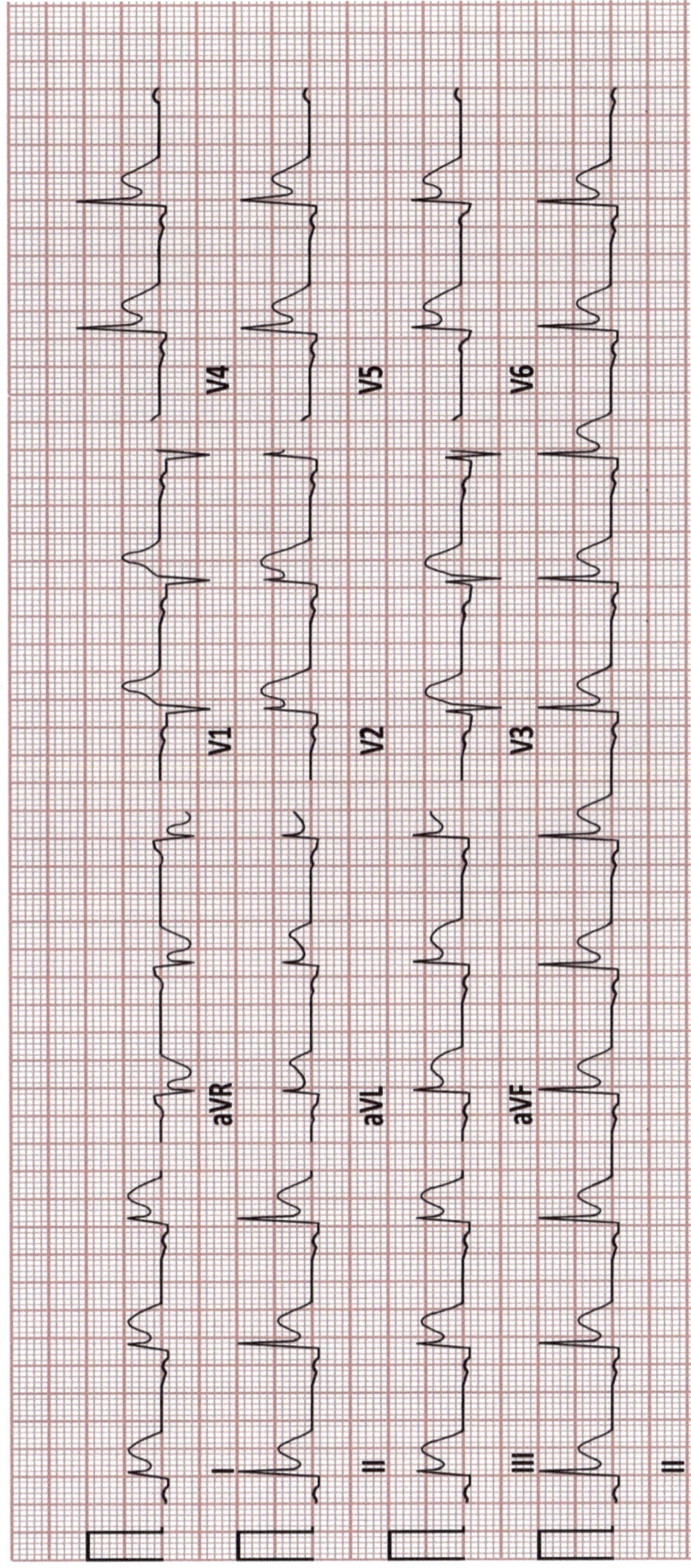

EKG Findings:
Rate: Normal
Rhythm: Regular
P wave: Normal
PR interval: Normal
QRS: Normal
+
Widespread ST elevation (diffuse ST elevation) **and PR segment depression**

ABBREVIATIONS AND SYMBOLS:

Abbreviation/ Symbols	Meaning
>	Greater than
<	Less than
≥	Greater than or equal to
≤	Less than or equal to
ACE I	Angiotensin-converting enzyme inhibitors
ACLS	Advanced Cardiac Life Support
A Fib	Atrial Fibrillation
A Flutter	Atrial Flutter
AMS	Altered mental status
AV node	Atrioventricular node
AVRT	Atrioventricular Re-entrant Tachycardia
AVNRT	Atrioventricular Nodal Re-entrant Tachycardia
BB	Beta-blockers
BP	Blood pressure
BPM	Beats per minute
CAD	Coronary artery disease
CABG	Coronary Artery Bypass Grafting
CCB	Calcium channel blockers
CKMB	Creatinine kinase myocardial band
COPD	Chronic obstructive pulmonary disease
EKG	Electrocardiogram
LOC	Loss of consciousness
MFAT	Multi-Focal Atrial tachycardia
MI	Myocardial infarction
NAC	Novel anticoagulant
NSTEMI	Non-ST Elevated Myocardial Infarction
PAC	Premature Atrial Contraction
PMI	Point of maximal impulse
PVC	Premature ventricular Contraction
SA node	Sinoatrial node
ST	Sinus Tachycardia
STEMI	ST Elevated Myocardial Infarction
SVT	Supraventricular Tachycardia
URTI	Upper Respiratory Tract Infection
V-Fib	Ventricular fibrillation
V-tach	Ventricular tachycardia
WPW	Wolff Parkinson White syndrome

INDEX

A
Advanced cardiac life support, 14, 15, 30, 31, 58, 59, 60, 61
Altered mental status 4
Amiodarone, 20, 21, 37
Angina
    Unstable, 69, 70
    Stable 69, 70
Angiotensin Converting Enzyme Inhibitors, 70
Apixaban, 21, 37
Asystole, 58
Atropine, 40, 42, 44, 46, 48
Atrial Fibrillation, 36
Atrial Flutter, 20
Atrioventricular Re-entrant Tachycardia, 18, 26
Atrioventricular Nodal Re-entrant Tachycardia, 18, 26
aVL, 68, 76
aVF, 68, 76

B
Beta blockers, 20, 21, 26, 37, 70
Blood pressure, 4, 12, 14, 30, 58, 60
Blood supply to heart, 66
Bundle of His, 6, 26
Bundle of Kent, 18

C
CABG (Coronary artery bypass graft), 70, 73
Calcium channel blocker, 18, 20, 21, 26, 37, 40, 42, 44, 46, 48
Cardiac Anatomy, 6
Cardiac Physiology, 7
Cardioversion 1, 4, 5, 15, 31, 59, 61
CHADS Score, 21, 37
Chronic obstructive pulmonary disease, 34, 50
Conduction system of the heart, 6
Congenital Long QT Syndrome, 54
Congestive heart failure, 21, 37
Coronary Artery Disease, 21, 37
Coronary Catheterization, 68, 73
Compression of the carotid sinus, 26
CPR, 15, 31, 59, 61
Creatinine kinase myocardial band (CKMB), 69, 70, 72, 73

D
Dabigatran, 21, 37

Delta wave, 18
Diabetes, 21, 37
Digoxin, 1, 18
Diltiazem, 20, 21, 26, 37

E
Electrical Alternans, 62
Epinephrine, 15, 31, 59, 61

F
First Degree Heart Block, 42

H
Hypercalcemia, 57
Hyperkalemia, 57
Hypertension, 21, 37
Hypocalcemia, 57
Hypokalemia, 57
Hypotension, 4, 14, 30, 58, 60, 62
Hypothermia, 56
Hypoxia, 50, 53, 60

I
Infarction, 14, 30, 40, 42, 69, 72, 76
Ischemia, 66, 67, 69, 76

L
Left anterior descending artery, 67, 68
Left circumflex artery, 67, 68
Loss of consciousness, 1, 14, 30, 54

M
Metoprolol, 20, 26, 37, 70
Multi-Focal Atrial Tachycardia, 34
Myocardial infarction, 14, 30, 40, 42, 66, 67, 68, 69, 70, 72, 76

N
Non-ST Elevated Myocardial Infarction, 69, 70
Novel anticoagulant, 21, 37
Nitroglycerine, 70, 72

O
Oxygen, 15, 31, 59, 61

P
Pacemaker, 44, 46, 48, 54
Pericarditis, 78
Point of maximal impulse (PMI), 62
Posterior descending artery 67, 68
Procainamide, 18
Premature Atrial Contractions, 52
Premature ventricular Contractions, 53
Propranolol, 54
Pulselessness, 14, 30, 58, 60
Pulseless Electrical Activity, 60

R
Rate, 10
Rhythm, 11
Right coronary artery, 67, 68
Rivaroxaban, 21, 37

S
Second Degree Type 1 Heart Block, 46
Second Degree Type 2 Heart Block, 48
Shockable, 15, 31, 59, 61
Sinus Bradycardia, 40
Sinus Tachycardia, 24
ST elevated myocardial infarction (STEMI), 72
ST depression, 69
ST elevation, 72
Stress test, 70
Stroke, 21, 37
Supraventricular Tachycardia, 26

U
Unstable patient, 4
Unconscious, 14, 30, 58, 60

T
Third Degree Heart Block, 44
Torsades de pointes, 28
Transesophageal echo, 20, 21, 37
Transient ischemic attack, 21, 37
Troponin, 69, 70, 72, 73

V
V1, 68, 72, 76
V2, 68, 76
V3, 68, 76
V4, 68, 76
V5, 68, 76
V6, 68, 72, 76
Vascular disease, 21, 37
Ventricular Fibrillation, 30
Ventricular Tachycardia, 14

W
Wandering Pacemaker, 50
Warfarin, 20, 21, 37
Wolff Parkinson White Syndrome, 18

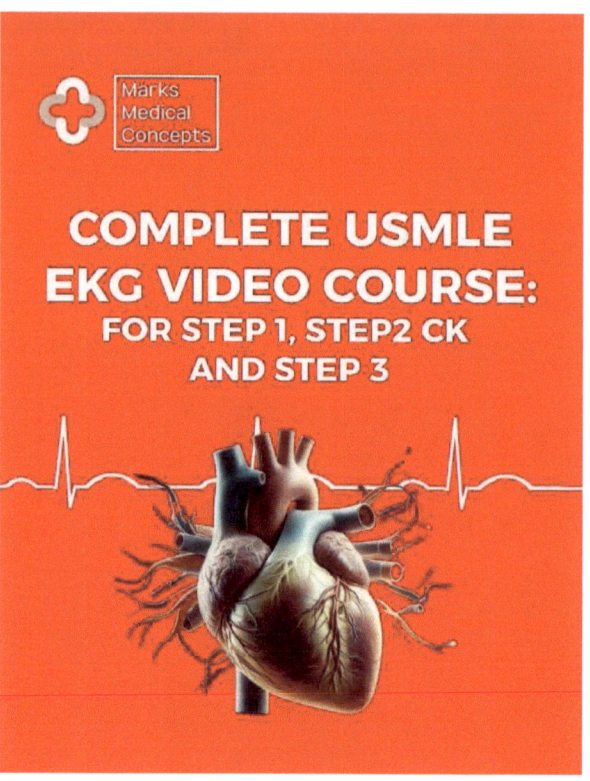

If you loved this book, check out our amazing concise video course:

COMPLETE USMLE EKG VIDEO COURSE

It is a great review resource before taking step 1, step 2 or step 3 exams and is definitely a course every one preparing for any exams needs to go through.

Sign up at:

www.marksmedicalconcepts.com/usmle